Advancing Responsible Adolescent Development

Series Editor
Roger J.R. Levesque
Indiana University, Bloomington, IN, U.S.A

More information about this series at http://www.springer.com/series/7284

Richard Jessor

The Origins and Development of Problem Behavior Theory

The Collected Works of Richard Jessor

Springer

Richard Jessor
Institute of Behavioral Science
University of Colorado at Boulder
Boulder, CO, USA

ISSN 2195-089X ISSN 2195-0903 (electronic)
Advancing Responsible Adolescent Development
ISBN 978-3-319-40885-9 ISBN 978-3-319-40886-6 (eBook)
DOI 10.1007/978-3-319-40886-6

Library of Congress Control Number: 2016946354

Printed on acid-free paper

This Springer imprint is published by Springer Nature
The registered company is Springer International Publishing AG Switzerland

For
Kim and Tom
Merce and Howie
and
Jane

Preface

This is the first of three volumes bringing together key publications—journal articles and book chapters—that have marked the development of Problem Behavior Theory from its early framing to the version of the theory that is applied in current research. The selections are those from a larger corpus of work that have advanced understanding of adolescence and adolescent health and development. Making them available in this way is, in part, a response to the numerous inquiries and requests that continue to arrive from researchers across the globe.

But my hopes for the volumes extend beyond the greater access they provide to what we have written over the nearly six decades of the theory's implementation. Perhaps most salient is my hope that this volume and the two that follow will serve to exemplify the role that *psychosocial theory* can play in providing coherence and cumulativeness and generality to social inquiry, the selections having been guided by the concepts and the logic of Problem Behavior Theory. My hope also is that the works collected in the volumes can make clear the advantage of transcending disciplinary boundaries, particularly those that enclose the disciplines of psychology and sociology, in order to encompass *both person and context* in efforts to understand young people's lives. And finally, the selections constitute, together, a body of replicated, evidence-based knowledge about a major social problem—adolescent risk behavior; my hope is that they can help inform social policy and practice in ways that reduce such behavior and enhance opportunities for positive youth development.

The primary aim of the selections in this first volume is to convey a sense of the dynamic evolution of a conceptual framework, Problem Behavior Theory, as it expanded its concerns from those it was initially designed to address. As successive research projects yielded their findings, they impelled us to modify the theory's structure and to extend its reach; this is the way science is supposed to work. The grasp that the earlier selections in the volume can provide about the origins of the theory should enable a deeper understanding of the current formulation of Problem Behavior Theory and of the breadth of its applications.

Volume II, *Problem Behavior Theory and Adolescent Health*, brings together key, theory-guided publications that, over the years, have examined the large variety of behaviors that can compromise adolescent and young adult health. The concept of "health" in that volume is broader than just physical health, i.e., morbidity and mortality. Rather, it engages all those behaviors that put an adolescent at risk and that can interfere with successful development into young adulthood. Scholars concerned with particular health-compromising behaviors, whether tobacco smoking or risky driving or early, unprotected sex or unhealthy diet or sedentariness, will find selections in that volume relevant to their interests. And in Volume III, *Problem Behavior Theory and the Social Context*, the selections are those that have shown the explanatory gain derived from engaging the social environment or the immediate context of action in research on adolescence and young adulthood. In addition, the third volume includes selections that articulate the philosophy of science perspective and the methodological posture that have threaded their way through all of the body of work presented in all three volumes.

In a scholarly journey over this long period of time, there has been the accumulation of a range of debts, both intellectual and interpersonal, that have helped to determine the direction of the journey and the contours it has traced. It is a distinct pleasure to acknowledge them here. First, the home base for my research since the late 1950s has been the Institute of Behavioral Science at the University of Colorado Boulder. Whether as one of the founders of the institute, as director of the institute for over two decades, or as founder of two of its research programs, my life has been endlessly enriched by interactions with its dedicated scholars and students intent on contributing to society's well-being. Ozzie G. Simmons, the institute's first full-time director in the early 1960s; Gilbert F. White, the institute director I succeeded in 1980; and Jane A. Menken, the institute director who succeeded me in 2001—all three have earned my appreciation for shaping the institute into the benign, supportive, and productive institution it has been. I am grateful to have had such a friendly and fertile environment in which to pursue my own line of scholarly inquiry.

Throughout my career, I have had exceedingly good fortune in collaborations with colleagues and students whose ideas informed my own and whose work is apparent in the selections in these volumes. Foremost among them is my first wife, Dr. Lee Jessor, who was in at the very beginning and whose contributions helped lay the foundation for what was to become Problem Behavior Theory. Among the many other collaborators, especially in the later years, Drs. John E. Donovan and Frances M. Costa, both my former students, and Mark S. Turbin deserve special tribute for their commitment to our research program, their ideas, and their hard work.

Appreciation also goes to the foundations and federal agencies that provided the funds that enabled us to undertake the complex, often time-extended research projects that undergird the selections in these volumes; special acknowledgment goes to the William T. Grant Foundation and the John D. and Catherine T. MacArthur Foundation and to the National Institute of Mental Health, the National Institute on Alcohol Abuse and Alcoholism, and the National Institute on Drug Abuse.

Publishing this corpus of work required a cohort of enablers over the decades. Special mention and much appreciation go to Marilyn Sena, Debbie Ash, Mary Axe, Steve Graham, Rajshree Shrestha, and now Nancy Thorwardson and Lindy Shultz, the latter two helping to bring these volumes into being.

Finally, it would be difficult to count all the ways in which my wife, Jane Menken, my companion in scholarship and adventure these past several decades, has influenced what I have sought to accomplish. That influence has been a gift that I continue to cherish.

Boulder, CO, USA Richard Jessor, PhD, ScD

Contents

About the Author

Richard Jessor, PhD, ScD is a distinguished professor of behavioral science and professor of psychology, emeritus at the University of Colorado Boulder where he has spent his entire academic career. One of the founders of the university's Institute of Behavioral Science in 1959, he served as its director from 1980 to 2001. He was the founding director of the institute's Research Program on Problem Behavior and, later, its Research Program on Health and Society. From 1987 to 1997, he also directed the MacArthur Foundation Research Network on Successful Adolescent Development Among Youth in High-Risk Settings. He is the author or editor of ten books and has published over 135 articles and book chapters. In 2003, he was designated as a "Highly Cited Researcher" in the Social Science General category by the Institute for Scientific Information.

Educated at the College of the City of New York and Yale University, where he received his B.A. degree in psychology in 1946, Jessor received an M.A. from Columbia University in 1947 and a Ph.D. in clinical psychology in 1951 from Ohio State University, where he was a student of Julian B. Rotter. He has been a consultant to various federal agencies and private foundations as well as the World Health Organization, Health and Welfare Canada, and UNICEF. He has served on several National Research Council panels and on the Carnegie Council on Adolescent Development. He was an invited fellow at the Center for Advanced Study in the Behavioral Sciences in 1995–1996, and he received the Outstanding Achievement in Adolescent Medicine Award in 2005 from the Society for Adolescent Medicine. Jessor is, after 65 years, the longest-serving active faculty member at the University of Colorado. In May 2015, he was awarded the degree of Doctor of Science, honoris causa, by the Regents of the University of Colorado.

Chapter 1
Introduction to the Volume

Richard Jessor

Introduction

The social–psychological conceptual framework known as Problem Behavior Theory continues to be widely used in contemporary research with adolescents and young adults. The theory, an evolving product of an effort initiated over a half century ago, is now a comprehensive, interdisciplinary, explanatory framework to account for variation in young people's behavior, health, and development.

Cited more than 25,000 times as of this writing by scholars across the globe, Problem Behavior Theory is currently relied upon not only in a variety of researches but also in the design of prevention/intervention programs for young people. How the theory originated, how it evolved and expanded beyond the problem behavior domain, how it has been transformed from its initial framing to its current version, and what its key contributions have been is what the chapters in this volume are about. Those chapters, taken together, constitute a definitive account of the present formulation of Problem Behavior Theory, as well as its explanatory reach.

The initial selection in this volume, Chap. 2, provides something of a "biographical" overview of the development of the theory—its ontogeny—from its earliest origins to its maturity in present-day applications. Throughout the nearly six decades of its development, the overriding objective has been to achieve an explanatory framework that could illuminate important societal problems, that encompassed both person and contextual variation, that could capture individual and social environmental change, and that linked logically and predictively to significant social behavior.

R. Jessor (✉)
Institute of Behavioral Science, University of Colorado at Boulder, Boulder, CO 80309, USA
e-mail: jessor@Colorado.edu

R. Jessor, *The Origins and Development of Problem Behavior Theory*,
Advancing Responsible Adolescent Development,
DOI 10.1007/978-3-319-40886-6_1

Achieving such an objective was elusive in the decade after the end of World War II. Most psychology departments in US universities were still dominated by an arid behaviorism based almost entirely on animal models of learning in laboratory experiments. Engaging with persons and their lives was usually limited to psychological clinic settings, and these were often dominated by psychoanalysis. Neither behaviorism nor psychoanalysis had room in its conceptual framework for the larger societal context, and neither viewed persons from the perspective of their social experience and social learning over the life course.

My own concern with social problems, and my life-long commitment to address them, emerged from exposure to Marxism and Marxist theory early in my high school years, exposure that intensified after high school in the heady political atmosphere that prevailed at the College of the City of New York where daily political debates among diverse factions of radical students often took precedence over attending classes. World War II interrupted that shaping experience but, serving as a Marine in combat on Iwo Jima, I personally experienced perhaps the most devastating of all social problems, and that only deepened my concern and strengthened my commitment. Post-war years finishing my B.A. degree in psychology at Yale and gaining an M.A. in psychology at Columbia were, from a perspective of concern for social problems, rather disappointing. At Yale, the behaviorism of Clark Hull's learning theory pervaded the course offerings while, at Columbia, it was Skinnerian behaviorism that influenced the departmental climate.

It was only when I arrived at The Ohio State University in 1947 for my doctoral training in clinical psychology that I encountered an atmosphere more compatible with my own enduring social concerns and commitments. The opportunity there to work with Julian B. Rotter who was in the process of formulating what became his social learning theory of personality (1954) opened up a window for me on theory development that viewed persons in social–psychological rather than psychoanalytic terms, that engaged their contexts of daily life—their social and psychological situations—and that, unlike the learning theories of Hull and Skinner, attended to their subjective awareness, especially their values and expectations and beliefs. The doctoral time with Rotter was formative, and his influence, which has had a lasting impact on all of my work, is most evident in how Problem Behavior Theory was initially formulated.

Initiating an Interdisciplinary, Social–Psychological Conceptual Framework

The conceptual framework that ultimately became Problem Behavior Theory was, as detailed in Chap. 2, constructed for what was called *The Tri-Ethnic Community Study*, a 1959–1962 research project originally funded to account for heavy alcohol use among Native Americans in a small community in the Rocky Mountain region. The community comprised Native Americans, long-time Spanish–American residents, and Whites or Anglos. It was immediately apparent to us from observations in the community that the tri-ethnic social context could not be ignored in any attempt to explain social behavior, deviant or otherwise, that it varied markedly across the three ethnic groups in the community, and that a psychological approach alone could not hope to provide an adequate explanatory account. That realization precipitated an extended effort, along with colleagues Lee Jessor, Theodore Graves, and Robert Hanson, to incorporate concepts from the social context disciplines—sociology primarily, especially Merton's (1957) concept of *anomie*, and also anthropology—as well as from psychology, in a novel, interdisciplinary, explanatory framework. That framework was the origin of what later became Problem Behavior Theory. Given the disciplinary parochialism and isolation of the time, the early 1960s, constructing a systematic interdisciplinary framework was, looking back, an audacious undertaking, a rather bold venture into what today might be called trans-disciplinary behavioral science.

Despite early trepidations about the interdisciplinary course we had embarked on, we were ultimately able to see that we had, indeed, pursued a fruitful strategy. In the end, our Tri-Ethnic Study findings revealed the explanatory power of the theoretical concepts in the framework; they were able to provide a compelling account of variation not only *between* the ethnic groups but also *within* each of the three ethnic groups. The book that emerged from this decade-long enterprise, Jessor, Graves, Hanson, and Jessor (1968) *"Society, Personality, and Deviant Behavior: A Study of a Tri-Ethnic Community,"* was well received and continues to be cited even today.

We had been given important encouragement a few years earlier when the initial chapters of the book were reviewed for the publisher in 1965 by the renowned social psychologist, Theodore M. Newcomb, at Michigan. He wrote that the chapter on "The Concept of Deviance": "…is a jewel. …I don't think I've seen a statement by a psychologist that is as sophisticated, sociologically. The detail and coherence of the three [theoretical] structures are novel, to my knowledge, and convincing—especially in research relevance."

Those remarks were an incentive for us to complete the manuscript for the volume, and we were subsequently gratified—and reassured—by the positive reviews the book received on its publication. The distinguished sociologist/criminologist, Solomon Kobrin, characterized the book as a "monumental work" and concluded his review by saying: "…this is a truly pioneering effort in the field of interdisciplinary behavioral research. The impressive accomplishment of the study has been to move the field off its long-time dead center of pious hope, speculative generality, and timid and inconclusive tests, into that moment of truth which comes only with commitment to rigorous research validation. With this study the prospects for fruitful cross-fertilization among the behavioral sciences have been vastly improved." (Kobrin, 1969, pp. 488, 490). Another reviewer commented that: "A significant feature of the book is the elegant theoretical framework…." The theoretical approach and the findings it generated in the Tri-Ethnic Study are summarized in Chap. 3.

The experience of carrying out the Tri-Ethnic Study impacted our subsequent work in several major ways. Perhaps the most important consequence was a strengthened commitment to theory and to theory-guided inquiry. It is unfortunate that so much of social science research, even today, is a-theoretical, merely descriptive, or simply exploratory and empirical. The likelihood of such efforts cumulating and yielding a corpus of findings that enhance understanding of complex social problems is limited. The grasp that theory provides on the underlying or causal influences determining social behavior is what enables findings to cumulate and permits generality of inference across descriptively different forms of behavior and different settings of action. It is theory that brings understanding to otherwise seemingly unrelated observations.

This strengthened reliance on theory was accompanied by a second impact, a deepened conviction that an understanding of social behavior can only be achieved by theory that encompasses *both* the person and the social context. Engaging context alone elides the individual variation that always obtains within every social context, and engaging persons alone elides the variation that always obtains between social contexts. Incorporation of both person and context attributes has characterized Problem Behavior Theory research ever since the Tri-Ethnic Study, whether context was assessed as perceived or was established objectively.

A third impact was renewed commitment to the methodological stance that Kurt Lewin had frequently articulated, namely, that theory could be tested not only in controlled experimental settings but also, and perhaps in a more ecologically valid way, in the very life contexts in which the phenomena of interest occur. In the Tri-Ethnic Study, we had been able to apply a methodological strategy of theory-derived and construct-validated measurement in multiple, converging studies in the very community setting in which the various behaviors of interest to us were occurring. The success of that study argued against the almost exclusive reliance on qualitative observation by social anthropologists and sociological ethnographers, as if that method alone was the exclusive approach mandated by the nature of community studies. Indeed, what the Tri-Ethnic Study showed was that theory-guided, *quantitative* inquiry could be carried out in the very complexity of community life, and that the results of such inquiry could be illuminating and compelling.

A fourth impact was a sharpened awareness that very different behaviors can achieve the same goals or serve the same or very similar purposes, and that a study initiated largely to explain heavy drinking had necessarily to attend to various other behaviors that might also be able to achieve the goals that motivated heavy drinking. In the Tri-Ethnic Study, that awareness led us to collect data on a large variety of normative transgressions, in addition to heavy drinking, and to test the explanatory framework against them, as well. Those tests suggested that there was, as anticipated, significant co-variation among the different behaviors, and this insight, in later work, yielded the novel and heuristic notion of a "*problem behavior syndrome*" about which more will be said later.

Fifth, the Tri-Ethnic Study made evident the contribution of personality concepts to an understanding of variation in social behavior. Despite a prevailing climate, at the time, of disenchantment with personality as conventionally measured, what the study showed was that personality characteristics *conceptualized at a social–psychological level*—as relatively enduring beliefs, values, and expectations—could provide a substantial account of variation in behavior, both deviant and conforming. Further, such personality measures also permitted an understanding of the individual differences that obtained among community members who occupied the very same position in society, i.e., the same socioeconomic status or the same ethnic group membership.

One other impact of the Tri-Ethnic Study is worth noting. When normative transgressions were the criterion to be explained, it was the concept of *controls*, both formal and informal and both social and personal, that emerged as most salient, and measures of controls tended to dominate the explanatory account. This finding about rules and regulation, important in its own right, also alerted us to the relevance of the distal–proximal distinction among variables in predicting a particular criterion measure, e.g., heavy drinking, in our case. A variable such as "high value on achievement" is distal from the criterion of heavy drinking since it does not itself implicate alcohol use; by contrast, a variable such as "peer models for drinking" is proximal to heavy drinking since it directly implicates alcohol use. A distal variable is linked to a criterion only by theory; while it thereby is expected to predict variation in heavy drinking, it is likely to be a weaker predictor than a more proximal variable that directly implicates that criterion. Understanding this distal–proximal dimension has enabled us to avoid the kind of misinterpretations, in some of the literature, about whether it is personality variables or environmental variables that are most important, or whether certain personality or environmental variables are more predictive than others. What is actually the case with many of these claims is that the variables that predict a criterion more strongly are usually those that directly implicate it, i.e., those that are more proximal to the criterion.

If sheer predictability is the goal, then proximal variables tend to do best, but if theory-testing is at issue, then the linkage of a theoretically specified distal variable, though possibly weaker, may be a more important and, indeed, more interesting outcome. What we learned about the general salience of our measures of the personal and social control variables in the Tri-Ethnic Study was that they were usually more proximal to the criterion predicted. In much of our subsequent Problem Behavior Theory research, we have repeatedly demonstrated that distal attributes, though nonobvious, though often far removed in the nomological network, and though linked only by theory to the criterion of interest, do contribute significantly—by virtue of the theory—to the explanatory account.

Seeking a Grasp on Psychosocial Growth and Developmental Change

Despite its accomplishments, the Tri-Ethnic Study had a major limitation with respect to causal inference: it was cross-sectional in design. Although the multiple, converging studies permitted strong inferences about relationships, they were unable irrefutably to disentangle directionality of influence. Nor could the cross-sectional design reveal the *course of psychosocial development* over time, the development of those attributes—personal, social, and behavioral—delineated in the theoretical framework. The inherent silence of the Tri-Ethnic Study about adolescent growth and development propelled us to undertake the next phase of our theory-guided program of inquiry—a *longitudinal* study of cohorts of young people. That next project, *The Socialization of Problem Behavior in Youth Study,* and its theory and findings are summarized in Chap. 4.

In designing the longitudinal study in close collaboration with Lee Jessor, a social–developmental psychologist, we had the opportunity to start with student samples in middle school, earlier in the life course than the high school adolescents in the Tri-Ethnic Study, and with college freshmen, later in the life course than the high school students in the Tri-Ethnic Study. The study of these samples over 4 successive years, beginning in 1969, yielded, together, coverage of the developmental span from ages 12 to 22, i.e., from early adolescence to early adulthood. Since our samples were much more homogeneous in societal position than those in the Tri-Ethnic Study, the theoretical framework was elaborated to capture the adolescent's *perceived environment* in addition to structural/demographic status. And since this adolescent phase of the life course was the time when a variety of normative transgressions first emerge, the measurement of adolescent behavior was enlarged to encompass a wide variety of problem behaviors including alcohol and drug use, sexual experience, and delinquency and, for the purpose of establishing discriminant validity, to include conventional behaviors such as academic achievement and church attendance, as well.

It was in this longitudinal study, that the concept of *problem behavior* was introduced to replace our earlier reliance on the concept of *deviance*, and usage of the concept of problem behavior has now become firmly established in the general adolescent literature. This new, less pejorative, term emphasized that problem behaviors are departures from the norms of the larger, conventional society; it thereby avoided the previously troublesome issue, with the deviance concept, of whether those same behaviors may actually be conforming to other norms, the norms of the peer group or the norms of other subgroups. The new concept of problem behavior referred to those normative departures that were defined as problems by the larger society, that were likely to elicit some form of sanctions, and that usually resulted in negative consequences or difficulties for the adolescent. It has turned out to be a salutary conceptual revision.

Although *The Socialization of Problem Behavior in Youth Study* was longitudinal in design, it nevertheless enabled tests of the revised Problem Behavior Theory's explanatory relevance at each of the four, annual cross-sectional data waves for both the middle school and the college freshmen samples, tests that further confirmed the ability of the theory to account for cross-sectional variation in adolescent problem behavior. It also provided convincing evidence that problem behaviors tended to co-vary in adolescence, and it generated the novel concept of a *problem behavior syndrome*. Later studies that focused on further establishing the syndrome and its importance are presented in Chaps 6 and 7. Our syndrome findings constituted a strong challenge to the hallowed tradition among researchers at that time of studying each adolescent problem behavior separately; unfortunately, that tradition of specializing in a particular problem behavior—alcohol use or drug use or sex—was largely a reflection of the separate NIH institutes, each only funding research on a particular problem behavior at that time, as if it occurred in isolation from others.

But the major aim of *The Socialization of Problem Behavior in Youth Study,* and perhaps its overriding contribution, was to illuminate *adolescent development* and the role played in developmental growth and change by engagement in problem behavior. The four annual waves of data collected made it possible to plot developmental curves of involvement in the various problem behaviors over that time period, as well as curves of developmental change in the explanatory variables—values, attitudes, and beliefs—in the theoretical framework. Those developmental curves were shown to be *theoretically* parallel, i.e., that while there was a general increase in involvement in problem behavior over the 4 adolescent years, that the changes in the explanatory variables over the same time period were in the theoretical direction predictive of that observed increase. The coherence of theoretically parallel developmental change in both the predictors and the criterion measures of problem behavior involvement provided important evidence of the developmental relevance of Problem Behavior Theory.

Also developmentally compelling were other analyses showing that measures of the theoretical variables obtained *prior to* the initial occurrence of particular problem behaviors—first drink, first use of marijuana, first sexual intercourse—could account for variation in the later time of onset of those behaviors, i.e., were predictive of whether initiation happened at an earlier or a later subsequent data wave. Chapters reporting several of these predictive studies of the timing of problem behavior onset are presented in Volume II (Jessor, forthcoming, *Problem Behavior Theory and Adolescent Health*). Our pursuit of this type of predictive research was animated by a novel theoretical concept that was first introduced in the *Socialization of Problem Behavior in Youth Study*, the concept of *transition proneness*. In our earlier, cross-sectional research, we employed the concept of *problem behavior proneness* to summarize the likelihood of engaging in problem behavior given the pattern of the measures in the explanatory framework. Our awareness that many of the problem behaviors were *age-graded*, that is, were no longer considered a normative transgression beyond a certain age or stage of development, and indeed, were seen by young people as markers of a more mature or more experienced status, led us to "translate" the cross-sectional concept of problem behavior proneness into the developmental concept of transition proneness. The transition proneness concept now summarized *the likelihood of making a developmental transition*, given the pattern of the measures in the explanatory framework, a developmental transition from abstainer to drinker, from virgin to non-virgin, from nonsmoker to smoker, i.e., from a less mature to a socially defined, more mature status.

These successful developmental applications of Problem Behavior Theory placed our work firmly within the developmental science of adolescence. An additional contribution of our work to that science may have been the perspective that, for the most part, engaging in problem behavior in adolescence was part of *normal development,* and that recourse to psychopathology or, more recently, to the so-called immature adolescent brain to explain adolescent problem behavior was generally inappropriate and gratuitous, if not also reductive.

The full report of *The Socialization of Problem Behavior in Youth Study* and of its cross-sectional and longitudinal findings was published as the book: Jessor and Jessor (1977). *Problem Behavior and Psychosocial Development: A Longitudinal Study of Youth.* We were pleased with the review that appeared in *Social Forces*: "The monograph is an important contribution to the social psychology of adolescence.

It is essential reading for scholars in adolescence, deviance, delinquency, and social psychology generally. Moreover, it is an exemplar for students in social and behavioral science of what theoretically grounded research can and should be" (Pratto, 1979, p. 1025). It has now been cited over 6000 times and has been referred to in the literature as the "classic" work on Problem Behavior Theory.

An Explanatory Foray of Problem Behavior Theory into Young Adulthood

With the book about problem behavior in the adolescent portion of the life course completed, we had the good fortune—and the rare opportunity—to follow up those same cohorts in adulthood, 7 years after the last wave of their adolescent information had been collected. *The Young Adult Follow-Up Study* was able to recontact over 90 % of the original middle school and college freshmen participants and to gain their renewed participation in a two-wave, longitudinal continuation of the study, now as young adults. By the time of the second young–adult data wave in 1981, the middle schoolers had reached the ages of 25, 26, and 27, and the college freshmen had reached the age of 30, a significant span of young adulthood. A summary of the theoretical framework and the findings of this transition-to-adulthood research project is presented in Chap. 5.

Of particular developmental interest was the degree of *continuity* the study revealed between the earlier adolescent phase of the life course and the later phase of young adulthood. Although a great deal of developmental change had taken place, in both problem behavior involvement and in the key theoretical attributes, between the two phases of the life course, there was considerable stability in those changes. Whether change was assessed by over-time stability coefficients or by the predictability of young adult problem behavior outcomes from measures taken earlier in adolescence, it was clear that involvement in problem behavior in adolescence and in young adulthood was correlated. This was the case even though involvement in problem behavior from late adolescence through young adulthood was on a declining trajectory, an actual reversal of the increasing direction that problem behavior involvement had taken within the adolescent years. What stability meant was that an adolescent who might have been heavily involved with problem behavior in adolescence and who decreased his or her involvement over the transition into young adulthood, nevertheless continued to maintain a higher level of involvement in young adulthood relative to others in the sample whose involvement also declined. The life course continuity that emerged from *The Young Adult Follow-Up Study* was suggestive of the notion of a *lifestyle*, a coherent organization of psychosocial and behavioral attributes that persists over time and circumstantial change.

The developmental decline in involvement in problem behavior with the transition to young adulthood was entirely consonant with the direction of the developmental changes in the theoretical predictors, almost all of which were now in the direction of increased conventionality. In much of the literature about problem behavior or delinquency, this developmental decline with entry into adulthood has been described as "maturing out," a consequence attributed in large part to entry into adult roles such as regular work or family and child rearing responsibilities. What *The Young Adult Follow-Up Study* contributed was insight into the changes in both personality and perceived environment attributes, that is, in the Problem Behavior Theory concepts that accompanied the so-called maturing out process or entry into adult roles.

The young adult follow-up research also enabled a determination of whether the problem behavior syndrome observed in adolescence was still apposite as a description of the structure of problem behaviors in young adulthood. As indicated in Chap. 5, problem behaviors among young adults do indeed co-vary and constitute a syndrome, just as was the case in adolescence. Chapters 6 and 7 present earlier reports that also confirmed the existence of a problem behavior syndrome. The demonstration of a problem behavior syndrome at both phases of the life course suggests the developmental persistence of a lifestyle established earlier in adolescence.

A final contribution of *The Young Adult Follow-Up Study* needing mention is the evidence it provided about consequences for young adulthood of having engaged, even heavily, in problem behavior, including heavy drug use, in adolescence. Across a variety of indicators in young adulthood, there was little evidence that engaging in problem behavior in adolescence had in any way mortgaged the adolescent's future. With regard to educational, work, or familial outcomes, there was no demonstrable variation attributable to earlier problem behavior involvement. Whether this was due to our samples being largely middle class, or to the fact that they were from a normal rather than a clinical population, or that what was defined as heavy involvement in our study was not extreme enough, the findings caution against claims of dire and lasting life consequences of adolescent involvement in problem behavior, claims issued by various interest groups including, unfortunately, certain government agencies.

Overall, *The Young Adult Follow-Up Study* helped establish a degree of *developmental invariance* of the Problem Behavior Theory account of problem behavior across the adolescence–young adulthood life span. The theoretical framework and findings of the study were published as: Jessor, Donovan, and Costa (1991). *Beyond Adolescence: Problem Behavior and Young Adult Development.* One reviewer, a leading sociologist, wrote of the book: "It is well known that longitudinal studies are rare in the social sciences. Longitudinal studies driven by a coherent conceptual framework, and competent, state of the art statistical analyses, are even rarer. Yet this is exactly what one finds in *Beyond Adolescence*....a major strength of this work is the merging of sociological and psychological concepts.... In my view, Jessor and his colleagues have enriched the behavioral sciences...." (Laub, 1993, pp. 408–409). Another reviewer, a well-known developmental psychologist, wrote: "On many counts, Jessor and his team were ahead of their time.... In sum, *Beyond Adolescence* demands careful study" (Cairns, 1995, pp. 1658–1659).

The three books reporting the findings of the three major studies, each summarized in Chaps. 3, 4, and 5, respectively, constitute a corpus of theory-guided, cross-sectional, and developmental research that was replicated across age groups, gender, and social settings. Together, they established the substantial contribution that

Problem Behavior Theory—a middle-range, interdisciplinary, explanatory framework—had made by the early 1990s to the understanding of an important social problem—problem behavior—in both adolescence and young adulthood.

Reformulating Problem Behavior Theory

In the 1980s, research guided by Problem Behavior Theory began to extend beyond the problem behavior domains in which it had traditionally been carried out, especially into the domain of adolescent health behavior. It had become evident that many of the problem behaviors we were studying, e.g., cigarette smoking, or unprotected sex, or risky driving, compromised adolescent health and were seen by health professionals not as problem behaviors but as *health* behaviors. It was also evident that various *non*-problem behaviors, e.g., unhealthy diet, sedentariness, and inadequate sleep, put an adolescent's health at risk. Both sets of behaviors posed risk to adolescent health and development and could, together, be characterized as *risk behaviors*. Since both sets of behaviors implicated norms, whether the norms of the larger society or those that were personal or endorsed by more immediate reference groups like family and friends, it seemed apparent to us that the theoretical framework of Problem Behavior Theory should prove relevant for an understanding of this larger category of adolescent risk behavior. It was that perspective that led to a reformulation of the concepts of Problem Behavior Theory into the risk factor and protective factor concepts employed in behavioral epidemiology.

In what has turned out to be an influential paper (Jessor, 1991), a comprehensive conceptual framework for the study of adolescent risk behavior and risk lifestyles was articulated (see Chap. 8). The framework illustrated the "translation" of concepts from Problem Behavior Theory into the language of risk factors and protective factors. Some examples: Low Self-Esteem in the Personality System and Models for Deviant Behavior in the Perceived Environment System were translated into or become risk factors; Intolerance of Deviance in the Personality System and Models for Conventional Behavior in the Perceived Environment System were translated into or become protective factors. In the reformulation, the psychosocial constructs that had been assessed in Problem Behavior Theory were conserved, but now were reorganized as psychosocial risk factors and protective factors, a language more accessible for those concerned with health. Protective factors were differentiated into: Models Protection, Controls Protection, Support Protection, and Behavior Protection; risk factors were also differentiated into four categories: Models Risk, Vulnerability Risk, Opportunity Risk, and Behavior Risk.

The reformulation, which is the contemporary structure of Problem Behavior Theory, had several salutary consequences beyond its ready accessibility for health professionals. It retained the theory's fundamental dialectic, previously between instigations and controls, now between risk and protection. It also made clearer the reliance of the theory upon the basic processes that undergird behavior and behavior change, i.e., the processes of social learning (here *modeling*), and both positive (here *supports*) and negative (here *controls*) reinforcement. And, in recognition of the moderating role that protection can have on the impact of exposure to risk, it transformed what was until then an additive model into one that is *interactive*, i.e., one that examines not only the direct effects of protection and of risk on behavior, but also the effect of the *protection-by-risk interaction*. The research studies reported in Chaps. 9, 10, and 11 in this volume exemplify the application of this protection/risk model of Problem Behavior Theory; they also illustrate the contribution that the interaction or moderator effect of protection on risk makes to the explanation of adolescent behavior and development. Various applications of the current model to the domain of adolescent health are presented in Chaps. 27, 28, and 29 in Volume II (Jessor, forthcoming, *Problem Behavior Theory and Adolescent Health*).

Establishing the Generality of Problem Behavior Theory

Two other directions pursued in Problem Behavior Theory research in the last couple of decades have enabled us to extend its reach into contexts of disadvantage and limited opportunity, on the one hand, and into contexts of cross-national variation, on the other. The findings from both these directions of inquiry have resulted in strengthening the claim of explanatory generality for Problem Behavior Theory. With regard to cross-national research, a longitudinal, comparative study of adolescents in Beijing, China, and in Denver at the turn of the century permitted a stringent test of the applicability of Problem Behavior Theory in a societal context that contrasted sharply with that of the USA on multiple, macro- and micro-dimensions. Despite these large contextual differences, and despite differences in mean levels of problem behavior in the two societies, the Problem Behavior Theory account of variation in problem behavior involvement was essentially invariant across both societies (see Chap. 10, this volume). Cross-national generality was further established in research on adolescents in the slums of Nairobi presented in Chaps. 4, 6 and 7 in Volume III (Jessor, forthcoming, *Problem Behavior Theory and the Social Context*). Various other investigators, e.g., Vazsonyi et al. (2010), have employed Problem Behavior Theory in studies in countries across the globe, and they have also extended and confirmed its applicability beyond the USA, the country in which the theory originated (see also Chap. 2, this volume, Part IV).

With regard to contexts of disadvantage and limited opportunity, Problem Behavior Theory research in such contexts began long ago, of course, with the *Tri-Ethnic Community Study*, but more recent studies were stimulated by my decade-long role as director of the MacArthur Foundation Research Network on Successful Adolescent Development among Youth in High Risk Settings (see Chaps. 2 and 5 in Volume III). The focus of that Network on how adolescents, confronting limited opportunity and scant resources, nevertheless manage to "make it," influenced our own efforts to apply Problem Behavior Theory in the social context of disadvantage, with both our Denver samples (see Chap. 3, Volume III) and our samples in the Nairobi slums (see Chaps. 6, 7, and 8 in Volume III). The illumination that Problem

Behavior Theory brought to adolescent behavior and development under conditions of adversity was convincing evidence of its generality across societal strata and differential access to opportunity.

The explanatory generality that these two directions of contextual research revealed derives from the fact that the inquiries were guided by theory. Theoretical concepts implicate underlying or causal processes rather than apparent, surface, or descriptive characteristics, and it is those underlying processes that are invariant across widely different contexts or settings (see Chap. 17 in Volume III).

Problem Behavior Theory and Non-Problem, Pro-Social Behavior

Finally, it is important to take note of the fact that Problem Behavior Theory has contributed to an understanding of *pro-social behavior and positive youth development*, as well. Insofar as the very name of the theory is about problem behavior, extending its reach into pro-social, conventional, or positive behavior warrants explanation. Throughout its development, however, Problem Behavior Theory research has, almost without exception, included measures of pro-social behavior such as school achievement, or church attendance, or civic engagement. This was motivated in part by a concern for discriminant validation, that is, by the need to demonstrate that those concepts in the theory that were positively related to problem behavior involvement were, at the same time, negatively, i.e., inversely, related to pro-social behaviors, and vice versa. The motivation was also to determine those Problem Behavior Theory attributes that could account directly, rather than by default, for variation in pro-social or positive behavior and development. Examples of the latter are such attributes as *value on achievement,* or *religiosity,* or *value on health*, attributes in the theory that reflect psychosocial conventionality and relate directly and positively to pro-social behavior involvement.

In the reformulated Problem Behavior Theory framework, the role of the protective factors—models, controls, and supports—is not only to protect against engaging in problem behavior, but also to *promote* pro-social, positive behavior. It is unfortunate that, in some of the recent literature on positive youth development, the almost exclusive emphasis on pro-social behavior in adolescence seems to have eclipsed any continued interest in problem behavior. Obviously, problem behavior and pro-social behavior can both be characteristics of the same individual, and a conceptual framework is needed that illuminates variation in both. The present protection-and-risk version of Problem Behavior Theory has already contributed in that regard (see Chap. 11, this volume). The research reported in Chap. 11 makes clear, for example, that different protective factors are engaged when accounting for problem behavior (largely Controls Protection) than when accounting for pro-social behavior (largely Models Protection and Support Protection). This is a novel contribution to the literature on positive youth development, and it testifies to the value of a comprehensive theory that encompasses both problem and pro-social behavior.

Conclusion

The chapters in this volume provide a window on the development of a psychosocial conceptual framework from its origin to its present, widely used formulation. As Problem Behavior Theory has evolved over more than half a century of applications, the explanatory account it has offered of adolescent and young adult behavior and development has been substantial. Equally impressive has been the robustness of its findings about problem behavior variation, findings robust across age, gender, socio-economic status, historical time, and even large cross-national differences. The knowledge generated about adolescent and young adult problem behavior, e.g., the critical role played by *both* person and contextual attributes; the *continuity* between the adolescent and young adult phases of the life course; the contribution of the *transition proneness* concept to predicting developmental change; the *syndrome* organization of problem behaviors in both adolescence and young adulthood; the *moderating role of protection* on the impact of exposure to risk; the *inverse relation* between problem behavior involvement and involvement in pro-social and health-enhancing behavior, suggesting the existence of a coherent *lifestyle*; and the *generality* that is the fruit of theory-guided research; all have helped to shape contemporary understanding of adolescence and young adulthood.

The research studies reported in this volume and in Volumes II and III enable, together, a strong claim on causal inference since they represent extended and cumulating *replications,* across adolescent development, across gender, across historical time, and across local, national, and international settings, of tests of theoretically specified relationships. The renowned methodologist, Jacob Cohen, has argued that: "A successful piece of research doesn't conclusively settle an issue.... Only successful future replication in the same and different settings...provides an approach to settling the issue" (Cohen, 1990, p. 1311). The style of Problem Behavior Theory social inquiry we have implemented over the decades has been fully consonant with that trenchant comment.

References

Cairns, R. B. (1995). Review of: *Beyond adolescence: Problem behavior and young adult development*, by Richard Jessor, John Edward Donovan, & Frances Marie Costa. *American Journal of Sociology, 100*(6), 1657–1660.

Cohen, J. (1990). Things I have learned (so far). *American Psychologist, 45*(12), 1304–1312.

Jessor, R. (1991). Risk behavior in adolescence: A psychosocial framework for understanding and action. *Journal of Adolescent Health, 12*(8), 597–605.

Jessor, R. (Forthcoming). *Problem Behavior Theory and adolescent health* (Vol. 2). New York: Springer.

Jessor, R. (Forthcoming). *Problem Behavior Theory and the social context* (Vol. 3). New York: Springer.

Jessor, R., Donovan, J. E., & Costa, F. M. (1991). *Beyond adolescence: Problem behavior and young adult development*. New York: Cambridge University Press.

Jessor, R., Graves, T. D., Hanson, R. C., & Jessor, S. L. (1968). *Society, personality, and deviant behavior: A study of a tri-ethnic community*. New York: Holt, Rinehart and Winston.
Jessor, R., & Jessor, S. L. (1977). *Problem behavior and psychosocial development: A longitudinal study of youth*. New York: Academic.
Kobrin, S. (1969). Review of: *Society, personality, and deviant behavior: A study of a tri-ethnic community*, by Richard Jessor, Theodore D. Graves, Robert C. Hanson, and Shirley L. Jessor. *Social Service Review, 43*(4), 488–490.
Laub, J. H. (1993). Review of: *Beyond adolescence: Problem behavior and young adult development*, by Richard Jessor, John Edward Donovan, & Frances Marie Costa. *Contemporary Sociology, 22*(3), 408–409.
Merton, R. K. (1957). *Social theory and social structure* (Rev. and enl. ed.). Glencoe, IL: Free Press.
Pratto, D. J. (1979). Review of: *Problem behavior and psychosocial development: A longitudinal study of youth*, by Richard Jessor & Shirley L. Jessor. *Social Forces, 57*(3), 1025–1026.
Rotter, J. B. (1954). *Social learning and clinical psychology*. Englewood Cliffs, NJ: Prentice-Hall.
Vazsonyi, A. T., Chen, P., Jenkins, D. D., Burcu, E., Torrente, G., & Sheu, C.-J. (2010). Jessor's problem behavior theory: Cross-national evidence from Hungary, the Netherlands, Slovenia, Spain, Switzerland, Taiwan, Turkey, and the United States. *Developmental Psychology, 46*(6), 1779–1791.

Chapter 2
Problem Behavior Theory over the Years

Richard Jessor

> A strong, overly zealous commitment to one's theory is important to scientific advancement.
>
> Donald T. Campbell

Part I

Introduction

It all started in 1958. An unexpected opportunity presented itself to become involved in a large-scale community study of an important social problem—alcohol abuse—in a marginalized group in American society, Native Americans. This chapter sketches the successive phases, from that point to the present, of the systematic development of Problem Behavior Theory, a theory increasingly employed in research on adolescent risk behavior by scholars in the USA and abroad. In a certain sense, the "biography" of that theory is the autobiography of my half-century of research and writing about the developmental science of adolescence.

In the time since my PhD in Clinical Psychology from Ohio State University in 1951, I had been teaching, doing clinical training, and conducting research studies with both college sophomores and laboratory rats at the University of Colorado.

Reprinted with permission from:
Jessor, R. (2014). Chapter 23: "Problem Behavior Theory: A half-century of research on adolescent behavior and development." In R. M. Lerner, A. C. Petersen, R. K. Silbereisen & J. Brooks-Gunn (Eds.), The developmental science of adolescence: History through autobiography (pp. 239–256). New York: Psychology Press.

R. Jessor (✉)
Institute of Behavioral Science, University of Colorado at Boulder, Boulder, CO, USA
e-mail: jessor@Colorado.edu

R. Jessor, *The Origins and Development of Problem Behavior Theory*,
Advancing Responsible Adolescent Development,
DOI 10.1007/978-3-319-40886-6_2

The reach of those activities was limited, and I was feeling disaffected about the current state of psychology and dispirited about the significance of my own classroom and animal studies. Psychology as a scientific discipline in the early 1950s was still struggling with the arid legacy of behaviorism which had banished subjectivity and meaning from consideration, while clinical work suffered from the general absence of socially relevant theory, relying instead on outmoded trait approaches or derivations from the formulations of psychoanalysis, both largely insensitive to the influence of the societal context on individual development and adaptation. Getting involved in the large-scale community study seemed a promising avenue to re-invigorate my scientific activity, to enlarge my conceptual perspective beyond the discipline of psychology alone, to make my research more socially relevant, and to be able to focus on complex social behavior of societal significance. I decided to pursue the opportunity, and I helped write a grant application to the National Institute of Mental Health (NIMH) that was successful: 5 years of support and $300,000—large for that time. It was in designing and carrying out that research that what was to become Problem Behavior Theory was initially conceptualized and subjected to empirical scrutiny.

My alienation from conventional, discipline-focused, behavioral research had been growing ever since graduate school, fueled in part by an enriching involvement at Ohio State with Julian B. Rotter and his Social Learning Theory (Rotter, 1954) with its cognitive-social concepts of expectations and values and its contextual focus on the *psychological* situation. After joining the faculty at Colorado, I found myself challenging the behaviorist philosophy of science still dominating psychology, and I published several pieces critical of that perspective (e.g., Jessor, 1956, 1958), Along with colleagues, I also helped organize a symposium at Colorado on "Contemporary approaches to cognition" (Gruber, Hammond, & Jessor, 1957), one of the earliest volumes contributing to the so-called "cognitive revolution" in psychology which was just beginning to replace the behaviorist paradigm. But I had not yet been able to undertake the kind of research that would enable me to implement an alternative approach to inquiry about complex, human, social action; that was the opportunity that materialized with the 1958 grant award from NIMH. We were funded to carry out what came to be called "The Tri-Ethnic Study," and along with a team of collaborators that included Lee Jessor, a developmental psychologist, Ted Graves, an anthropologist, and Bob Hanson, a sociologist, we published our findings 10 years later in the volume *Society, personality, and deviant behavior: A study of a tri-ethnic community* (Jessor, Graves, Hanson, & Jessor, S.L., 1968). The social-psychological formulation of Problem Behavior Theory was first elaborated in that volume.

It seemed clear to me at the outset, in considering the opportunity provided by the NIMH grant award to undertake an alternative approach to social inquiry, that there would be a need to develop a coherent social-psychological theory, one that was problem-rather than discipline-focused (Kurt Lewin had long argued that basic research could, indeed, be accomplished in the context of studying applied problems). The theory would need to be multi-disciplinary, engage both person and environment, incorporate the perceived or phenomenal environment as well, and be attentive to the functions and goals of socially learned behavior. An ambitious and daunting agenda for a young scholar, to say the least!

In hindsight, I can think of three other important influences that helped to shape that agenda, beyond my felt disaffection with conventional psychological inquiry. First, I had been invited to spend the summer of 1954 as a member of a Social Science Research Council Interdisciplinary Summer Seminar on the topic of "occupational choice," along with two labor economists, two sociologists, and one other psychologist. The intense daily interaction across those summer months with colleagues from different disciplines—all of us intent on bringing understanding to such a complex, life-course process—taught me not only how to think beyond disciplinary boundaries, but the value and illumination of doing so. It had also provided me with the experience, for the first time, of delineating an interdisciplinary conceptual framework that incorporated, in logical fashion, constructs from the three disciplines involved. We published an integrative paper from that summer's work: "Occupational choice: A conceptual framework," (Blau, Gustad, Jessor, Parnes, & Wilcock, 1956).

A second major influence during the years leading up to the 1958 NIMH grant award was the formal establishment, in 1957, of the Institute of Behavioral Science on the University of Colorado campus, with participation of faculty and graduate students from multiple social science departments—anthropology, economics, political science, psychology, and sociology. Its establishment was the outcome of a growing recognition on the campus not only of the limitations of disciplinary research on human problems but of the explanatory benefits of transcending disciplinary boundaries. Having been an active participant in the deliberations and organizational planning that led up to our founding of the Institute, I was again exposed to the demands of interdisciplinary thinking and engaged again in cross-disciplinary interaction.

The third influence came from an enlarged understanding of the critical role of *theory* in guiding the research process and interpreting its findings. In my own field of personality research, much of measurement was employed opportunistically, relying on available instruments usually derived from popular views of personality variation, e.g., measures of introversion-extraversion. With the emergence, however, of attention to the requirements of "construct validity" (Cronbach & Meehl, 1955), the explanatory importance of deriving measures from theory, measures that represented the logical properties of the constructs they were intended to assess, became salient. A critique of the widely used Taylor Anxiety Scale, challenging its lack of construct validity (Jessor & Hammond, 1957), had required extensive exploration of the nature of theory in the philosophy of science literature and of the role that an explicit nomological network plays in measurement and explanation. That experience, coupled with my earlier involvement in Rotter's theory-building efforts while I was still a graduate student at Ohio State, and my later participation in developing the occupational choice conceptual framework, all combined to reinforce an enduring commitment to engaging theory in social inquiry.

Together, these influences resulted in what I would now recognize as a "developmental readiness," after 7 years of conventional research, to undertake the kind of challenge that the Tri-Ethnic Study presented, and to make a "developmental transition" to what seemed to me then to be a new, socially meaningful, and conceptually more comprehensive kind of research. It turned out to be a life- and career-changing transition that, I'm happy to say, is still reverberating.

Constructing Problem Behavior Theory for "The Tri- Ethnic Study": The Initial Formulation

Although the original concern of NIMH was with understanding Native American alcohol abuse, it was the case that the rural community in southern Colorado in which the research was to be carried out was actually tri-ethnic in composition, made up not only of Native Americans, but of historically long-settled Hispanic residents, and of Whites or, as they were called then, "Anglos." The possibility of designing a *comparative* study of the three ethnic groups living in the same small community, rather than focusing solely on the Native American population, was methodologically attractive: It could make clear whether there were factors influencing Native American drinking behavior that were, indeed, unique to them or shared by the other two groups. Further, although the concern of NIMH was with excessive alcohol use, it was quite obvious that alcohol abuse was generally associated with a range of other normative transgressions, some of which, upon analysis, were oriented to similar goals or served functions similar to those that drinking behavior served, and which might, therefore, have similar determinants. Thus, it seemed theoretically important to cast a wide measurement net that assessed other problem behaviors, e.g., crime and violence, in addition to drinking, and—for construct validity purposes—that also assessed conforming or conventional behaviors, like church attendance and, for adolescents, school achievement and school club involvement.

The primary task confronted was to conceptualize the social environment and the person in terms that implicated each other and that were, at the same time, relevant to variation in problem behavior. That is, the task was to construct what Merton (1957) had termed a "theory of the middle range," a theory relevant to a circumscribed domain of social action—in this case, problem behavior—and that can guide empirical inquiry, rather than a "grand" theory of the sort that had, in the past, characterized so much of sociology (e.g., Parsons, 1937) and psychology (e.g., Hull, 1943; Skinner, 1938).

Conceptualizing the Social Environment. Extensive exploration of the sociological and criminological literature, on the one hand, and intensive ethnographic experience in the tri-ethnic community, on the other, led to the conceptual differentiation of the social environment into three major structures of societal influence on the likelihood of occurrence of problem behavior—an *opportunity structure,* a *normative structure,* and a *social control structure*—with variables in each structure having directional implications for the occurrence/non-occurrence of problem behavior. Limited access to societally valued goals in the opportunity structure was posited to constitute *instigation or pressure* to engage in illegitimate means, i.e., in deviant or problem behavior, in order to achieve those goals. Greater exposure to dissensus in the normative structure—lack of agreement on appropriate ways of behaving, i.e., anomie—was posited to constitute *low normative control* against engaging in problem behavior; and greater access to engaging in problem behavior in the social control structure was posited to constitute *attenuated social control* against problem behavior.

The balance of instigation and controls at any given location in society was hypothesized to determine the *rates or prevalence* of problem behavior at that location. From this theoretical perspective, differences in problem behavior among the three ethnic groups in the community would be due to differences in their positions in those three social environment structures. The indebtedness of this social environment formulation to the seminal contributions of Merton's concept of "anomie" (1957) and Cloward and Ohlin's notion of "differential access to illegitimate means" (1960) is apparent and was gratefully acknowledged.

Conceptualizing the Person. Although the social environment formulation could provide a grasp on the social determinants of between-group differences in levels or rates of problem behavior, it could not provide an account of the *intra*-group variation that exists at every social location; in order to achieve the latter, an *individual-level* account, a formulation about *persons,* was required. For conceptualizing person-level influences on the likelihood of occurrence of problem behavior, we sought structures of cognitive-social variables that could be seen as logically related to the social environment structures, i.e., as their conceptual analogues at the individual level. The value and expectancy concepts in Rotter's Social Learning Theory appeared to be apposite; "value-expectancy disjunction" at the person level was seen as analogous to limited access to societally valued goals in the opportunity structure and constituted, therefore, a *perceived opportunity structure* in the person. In the same vein, cognitive-social variables, such as "belief in internal versus external control," and "alienation," constituted a *personal belief structure*, analogous to the normative structure at the social environment level. Finally, variables like "attitudinal intolerance of deviance" constituted a *personal control structure* to serve, at the person level, as an analogue of the social control structure in the social environment.

The resultant of these conceptualizations was a sociocultural environment system of structures of variables relevant to problem behavior and a personality system of structures of variables relevant to problem behavior that, together, could account for *between-group variation* as well as *within-group variation* in problem behavior. The initial conceptual framework of Problem Behavior Theory for the Tri-Ethnic Study is presented in Fig. 2.1 (Jessor et al., 1968, p. 132).

Collecting the Tri-Ethnic Study Data. Interview and questionnaire measures of each of those variables were developed from the logic of their properties, i.e., from a construct validity perspective, and they were then employed in three converging studies carried out in the community, all testing the theory: (1) a stratified, random household interview survey of the adults in the three ethnic groups in the community—the Community Survey Study; (2) an in-school questionnaire study of all the adolescent students attending the community high school—the High School Study; and (3) an interview study of a random sub-sample of the parents of the high-school students who had participated in the questionnaire study—the Socialization Study. Our aim in mounting three converging studies on independent samples was to be able to minimize inferential ambiguity and to make a more compelling test, in an actual, complex field setting, of our social-psychological theory of problem behavior.

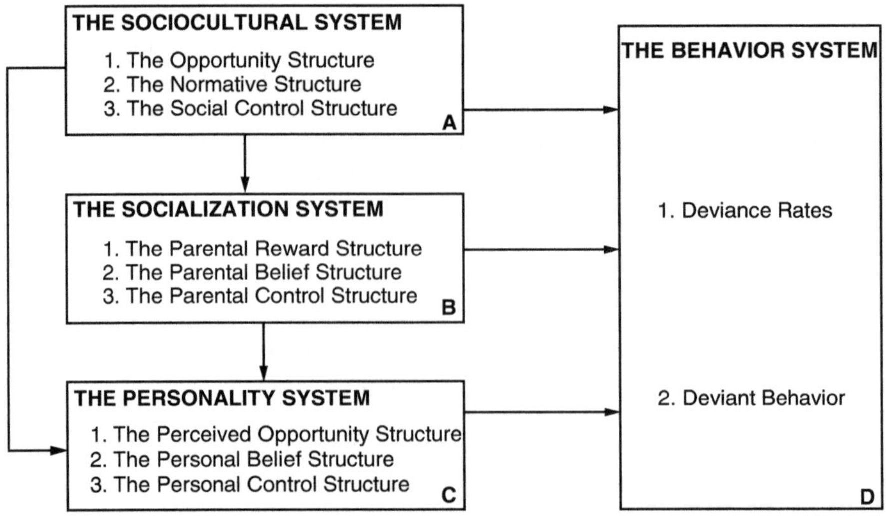

Fig. 2.1 The over-all social-psychological framework for the study of deviance (Jessor et al., 1968, p, 132)

That the theory was an effective guide for research was evident in the consonant findings from all three studies. Theoretical predictors from both the sociocultural system and the personality system, taken together, yielded a substantial account of problem behavior variation. Those findings held across the three ethnic groups and across gender, as well. Overall, results were as theoretically expected, and they provided strong encouragement for our conceptual labors.

Revising Problem Behavior Theory for "The Socialization of Problem Behavior in Youth Study": The Intermediate Formulation

The publication in 1968 of *Society, Personality, and Deviant Behavior: A Study of a Tri-Ethnic Community*, reported the first phase of the development of Problem Behavior Theory. My responsibility for that long-drawn-out enterprise definitively shaped the contours of my academic scholarship from that time forward. The 10 years of collaborative, interdisciplinary effort had been successful, the theory had been shown to be useful, the findings were illuminating, and the volume was well-received and, indeed, continues to be cited more than four decades later. An institutional outcome of the Tri-Ethnic research effort was the establishment, in 1966, in our Institute of Behavioral Science, of the interdisciplinary Research Program on Problem Behavior of which I became the founding director.

Despite its many strengths, however, particularly the conceptual mapping of both the social environment and the person in analogous terms relevant to problem behavior variation, and the theoretical coherence of the findings of its three converging studies, there was a fundamental shortcoming to the Tri-Ethnic work, namely, *it was cross-sectional in design.* The absence of time-extended data precluded inferences about causal direction or impact; remedying that limitation would require undertaking social inquiry that was *longitudinal* in design and that permitted the following of lives across extended and developmentally significant periods of the life course. An additional shortcoming was that, in assessing adolescents already in high school, it had elided the earlier adolescent life stage, a stage in which significant transitions occur or are prepared for. What seemed essential for a fuller grasp on adolescence was theory-guided longitudinal research that started earlier in the life course. A focus on the adolescent life stage and on adolescent behavior and development seemed the natural direction to pursue for the next stage of inquiry and for the further development of Problem Behavior Theory.

Even before the Tri-Ethnic book reached publication, however, a 1965–66 NIMH fellowship award enabled me to spend a full year learning about longitudinal research at the Harvard-Florence Research Project in Firenze, Italy, a unit that had been following three cohorts of boys since their early adolescence. The families of the boys all had their origin in southern Italy or Sicily, but the families of one cohort had migrated to Rome, the families of the second cohort had emigrated to Boston, and the families of the third cohort had remained in place. The year was extremely valuable for gaining a better understanding of how to follow young lives; it also provided an opportunity to interact with thoughtful developmental colleagues like Klaus Riegel and Douglas Heath, also resident that year at the Project, and it permitted me to carry out an interesting, cross-national, comparative study of drinking behavior in the three cohorts using selected psychosocial and behavior measures from Problem Behavior Theory (Jessor, Young, Young, & Tesi, 1970).

Armed with this experience, and in close collaboration with Lee Jessor, we began to plan a new longitudinal project that, while building on the accomplishments of the Tri-Ethnic Study, would revise and extend the theory to focus now on the behavior and development of young people during the entire adolescent stage of the life course. Two complementary, longitudinal studies of adolescents were designed, one beginning with middle-school adolescents, to be followed over four successive years (called the High School Study), and one beginning with college freshmen also to be followed over four successive years (called the College Study). Together, the two 4-year studies would span an age range from about 12 to 22, i.e., from early adolescence to late adolescence/early adulthood.

The cohort-sequential design for the middle schoolers involved lengthy, theory-derived questionnaires administered in school to initial samples of 7th-, 8th-, and 9th-grade students in the spring of each of the 4 years of the study, 1969–72, at the end of which they would be in 10th, 11th, and 12th grades, respectively. The simple longitudinal design used with the college freshmen also involved lengthy questionnaires administered in each of their four successive college years, 1970–73, at the end of which most would be in their senior year of college. Since this research took place at the end of the turbulent sixties and into the turmoil of the early seventies, the questionnaires included extensive sections on a variety of adolescent problem behaviors, including marijuana use, other, so-called "hard," drug use, alcohol use, delinquency, and for the first time, sexual activity, and also participation in militant protests; it also assessed involvement in a variety of conventional or pro-social behaviors, including academic effort and religious activity. The High School Study and the College Study were designed to permit testing Problem Behavior Theory cross-sectionally and longitudinally, and at earlier and later adolescent life stages. Unlike the tri-ethnic community, the setting for this proposed longitudinal study was a southwestern, largely White, middle-class, university community and its surrounding small towns, with only modest ethnic variation.

An application to NIMH in 1968 for support of a longitudinal project entitled, "The Socialization of Problem Behavior in Youth," was successful and, with later sponsorship by the National Institute on Alcohol Abuse and Alcoholism (NIAAA), yielded 7 years of funding. With the initiation of this new study, the second phase of the development of Problem Behavior Theory began. Nine years later, we published its findings in the volume *Problem, behavior and psychosocial development: A longitudinal study of youth* (R. Jessor & S.L. Jessor, 1977).

Conceptualizing the Perceived Environment. As with the Tri-Ethnic Study, the challenge was again to construct a theory of both the social environment and the person that had logical implications for the occurrence of, and intensity of involvement in, problem behavior. Given the relatively homogeneous nature of the new research community in terms of socio-economic status and ethnicity, and given that the focus was to be on adolescents, it seemed most informative in this study to explore and articulate the *perceived* environment rather than the social structural environment, as had already been done successfully in the Tri-Ethnic Study, The perceived environment is the environment as the adolescent sees it, the social environment that has meaning for the young person, an environment more proximal to action than the so-called "objective," social structural environment, and one that is consonant with such widely used concepts as "definitions of the situation" in sociology (Thomas, 1928) and "life space" (Lewin, 1935), "meaningful environment" (Rotter, 1954), and "phenomenal field" (Rogers, 1959) in psychology (for more on the perceived environment, see R. Jessor & S.L. Jessor, 1973). In this study, the social structural environment was dealt with in the more traditional way, i.e., demographically rather than conceptually, with several indicators of socioeconomic status and family structure employed largely as analytic controls.

The perceived environment, then, is the environment the adolescent—placed by the questionnaire in the role of quasi-ethnographer—perceives about parents and friends and peers and teachers, their support and controls and influence, and their acceptance/non-acceptance of problem behavior. It was differentiated into a *proximal structure,* with variables that directly implicate problem behaviors, e.g., having friends who model problem behavior, and a *distal structure,* with variables whose link to problem behavior is indirect and follows only from the logic of the theory, e.g., parental support. Although proximal variables generally relate more strongly to problem behavior outcomes, such relationships are obvious and less interesting theoretically than the relations of distal variables which derive from and can strengthen theory.

Conceptualizing the Person. The personality system for this project was delineated in essentially the same way as it had been for the Tri-Ethnic Study, with three structures of cognitive-social variables: one, the *motivational-instigation structure,* again mapped instigation or pressure to engage in problem behavior; and two, the *personal belief structure* and the *personal control structure*, again mapped controls against engaging in problem behavior. The measures employed were largely adapted from those devised for the earlier Tri-Ethnic Study, except for several new ones, such as a measure of social criticism, which was relevant to the new concern with militant protest behavior.

Shown in Fig. 2.2 (from R. Jessor & S.L., Jessor, 1977, p. 38), the conceptual framework encompasses both an environment system and a personality system, as it did in the Tri-Ethnic Study, as well as a comprehensive behavior system, the latter with both a *problem behavior structure* and a *conventional behavior structure.* (As the figure shows, and as was the case with the Tri-Ethnic Study, there was also an effort to study various socialization processes as influences on adolescent behavior and development.) Despite revisions of the theory, the basic Problem

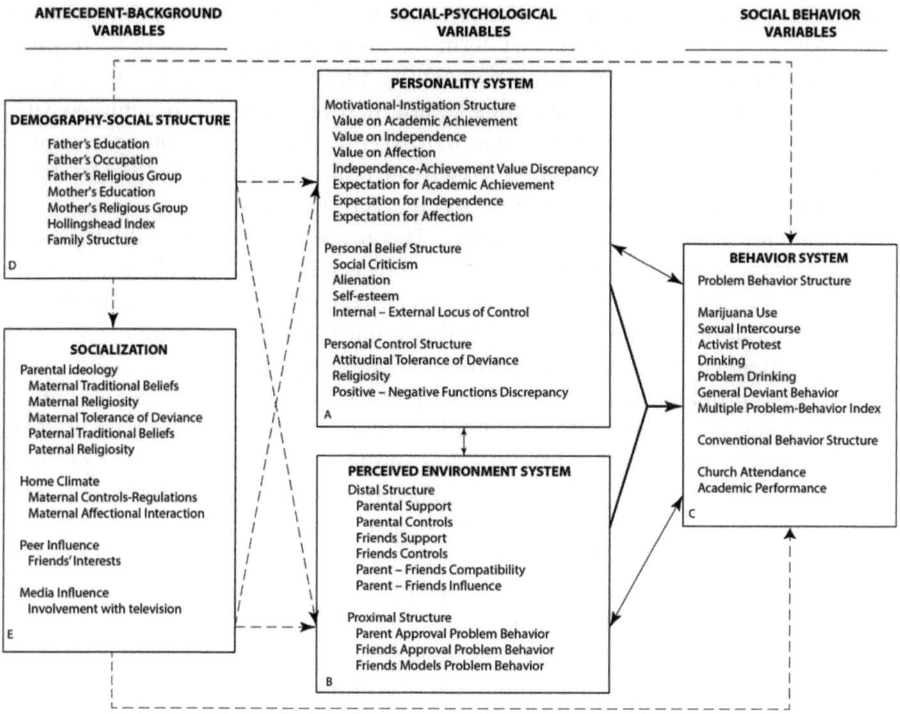

Fig. 2.2 The conceptual structure of Problem Behavior Theory (R. Jessor, & S.L. Jessor, 1977, p. 38)

Behavior Theory hypothesis remained the same: *Variation in the personality system and variation in the perceived environment system should each account for variation in problem behavior and, taken together, should provide a stronger account than either alone.* That hypothesis was tested in the two independent studies, the High School Study and the College Study, with both the cross-sectional data collected annually over the 4 years, as well as with the 4-year longitudinal data on each adolescent or young adult participant. Overall, the findings were impressive in their support of this later version of Problem Behavior Theory, the so-called "classical" version, published in the 1977 volume (for additional summary descriptions, see Costa, 2008; Donovan, 2005). In the cross-sectional analyses, the theoretical account of variance in problem behavior was substantial, as much as 50% for some of the problem behaviors; in addition, the personality and perceived environment predictors were inversely related to the conventional or pro-social behaviors, demonstrating discriminant validity; and finally, the findings, though based on local samples in a particular local setting, were supported by a national sample survey of 13,000 high-school youth carried out about the same time that employed a number of our Problem Behavior Theory measures (Donovan & Jessor, 1978; Jessor, Chase, & Donovan, 1980; Rachal, Williams, & Brehm, 1975). From the cross-sectional findings alone, it was clear that Problem Behavior Theory provided a useful grasp on variation in adolescent problem behavior in both the High School Study and the College Study.

The research also generated several important problem behavior concepts that have since entered the literature. The concept of *problem behavior proneness* was employed as a theoretical summary term for the likelihood of engaging in problem behaviors, based on the set of personality variables and the set of perceived environment variables that, theoretically, are their predictors. It became possible to think of *personality proneness*, and *perceived environment proneness*, as well as overall *psychosocial proneness,* based on both systems of predictors taken together. Another important concept that emerged from this inquiry was the *problem behavior syndrome* in adolescence. The research provided consistent evidence that there was co-variation or co-occurrence among very diverse problem behaviors, i.e., that various problem behaviors were inter-related and tended often to have similar determinants and to fulfill similar functions. The notion of a *syndrome* challenged the allocation to different Federal agencies of responsibility for the separate problem behaviors—thereby partitioning the "wholeness" or integrity of adolescent behavioral individuality—and it highlighted the parochialism of the research tradition that focused on a single or isolated adolescent problem behavior alone. The concept of a problem behavior syndrome has since generated an outpouring of adolescent research that is still underway; a recent review for the National Academies of Science of the cumulated research on covariance of problem behaviors in adolescence musters persuasive support for the syndrome concept (Monahan & Hawkins, 2012),

While the cross-sectional findings were gratifyingly consonant with those of the Tri-Ethnic Study of high-school youth, the overriding concern of this later longitudinal inquiry was to examine the reach of the theory in accounting for *developmental change* across adolescence and into early adulthood. Toward that end, both descriptive and predictive analyses were undertaken with the longitudinal data.

For the descriptive analyses, longitudinal "growth curves" were plotted across the 4 years of data, not only for the various problem behaviors, but also for their personality and perceived environment predictors. Beyond intrinsic interest in the developmental change that the curves documented on those attributes across four data points, they also revealed a *theoretical consonance of developmental change* between the behaviors and their predictors over time, constituting an initial, although indirect, test of the developmental usefulness of Problem Behavior Theory. For example, in the High School Study, value on academic achievement declined significantly over the 4 years of measurement, value on independence increased, and intolerance of deviance decreased among the personality system predictors; among the perceived environment system predictors, parental controls decreased, while friends models for drinking increased. Each of these directions of developmental change is theoretically predictive of a developmental *increase* in problem behavior over the 4 years of measurement, and, indeed, that was the case for marijuana involvement and for delinquent behavior, among others. Further, they are consonant with a *decrease* in conventional behavior which was the case for the measure of church attendance. This theoretical consonance of parallel developmental changes in adolescence of both predictor and criterion measures was a novel developmental finding, one that was supportive, indirectly, of Problem Behavior Theory.

A more direct test of the usefulness of the theory in accounting for developmental change in adolescence entailed predicting differences in time of onset of problem behaviors hitherto never engaged in. These analyses generated another important new concept, namely, the concept of *"transition proneness."* It was evident that, for many young people, engaging in problem behaviors such as drinking or smoking or having sex was a way of lodging a claim on a more mature status, i.e., of making a developmental transition. Since problem behaviors such as drinking or smoking or sexual intercourse are actually *age-graded behaviors*—behaviors that, while normatively proscribed for younger ages, are permitted or even prescribed for older ages, engaging in them for the first time can be a way of transgressing a norm, in this case an age norm, and thereby demonstrating that one is no longer a "kid." Problem Behavior Theory is designed to account for normative transgressions; that account should also apply to age norms, and the concept of "problem behavior proneness" therefore translates into or maps onto the developmental concept of "transition proneness," the likelihood of engaging in a transition-marking behavior. A number of tests of the notion of transition proneness were carried out in the High School Study where there were adequate samples of adolescents who had not yet initiated the problem behavior. What they demonstrated was the usefulness of the Problem Behavior Theory concept of transition proneness for predicting earlier versus later transition in regard to the onset of drinking, of marijuana use, and of becoming a non-virgin (Jessor, 1976; Jessor, 1987a; R. Jessor, Costa, S.L. Jessor, & Donovan, 1983; R. Jessor & S.L., Jessor, 1975; R. Jessor, S.L. Jessor, & Collins, 1972; S.L. Jessor & R. Jessor, 1975).

Overall, the longitudinal findings provided strong support for the developmental relevance of Problem Behavior Theory. They illuminated the developmental changes in those psychosocial attributes associated with, predictive of, and consequential upon the onset of transition behavior.

Extending Problem Behavior Theory Beyond Adolescence: "The Young Adult Follow-Up Study"

When the findings from the "Socialization of Problem Behavior in Youth Study" were published in the 1977 volume *Problem behavior and psychosocial development,* the second major phase in the evolution of Problem Behavior Theory came to a close. The High School Study and College Study participants, by the end of the longitudinal study in 1972 or 1973, respectively, had reached the ages of 16, 17, and 18 for the former, and 22 for the latter. To our great good fortune, the study of those same adolescents and young adults was to continue well into adulthood and to provide us with a unique opportunity to examine the applicability of Problem Behavior Theory to that later stage in the life course—young adulthood. With funding from NIAAA for "The Young Adult Follow-Up Study," we were able to launch a two-wave follow-up of our participants in 1979 and 1981; by 1981, the High School, Study youth had reached the ages of 25, 26, and 27, and the College Study youth had reached the age of 30, all having navigated the transition to adulthood. The findings from this longitudinal inquiry about problem behavior in adulthood were published in the volume *Beyond adolescence: Problem, behavior and young adult development* (Jessor, Donovan, & Costa, 1991), the third volume in the evolution and appraisal of Problem Behavior Theory.

In the interval since the fourth wave of data had been collected in 1972 and 1973, the longitudinal participants in our "Socialization of Problem Behavior in Youth Study" had scattered across the state, the nation, and even abroad. Locating them for follow-up was the initial challenge for the "Young Adult Follow-Up Study," a challenge that was met with extraordinary success: Almost all were located despite the significant passage of time, and fully 94% of both the High School longitudinal sample and the College longitudinal sample resumed their participation. Nearly all were out of school, most of the men and over half of the women were employed full-time, over half were married or in a committed relationship, and almost a third were raising families-evidence of the pervasive occupancy of the various roles of young adulthood. The two waves of data collected in 1979 and 1981 enabled examination of the usefulness of Problem Behavior Theory in accounting for variation in problem behavior *within* young adulthood, and they also enabled exploration of developmental change *between* adolescence and this later time in the life course.

Several important contributions to developmental science emerged from this extended appraisal of Problem Behavior Theory. First, variance accounted for in problem behavior in young adulthood was as substantial as it was in adolescence—mostly better than 40%, but with some exceptions for particular problem behaviors—in both the 1979 and the 1981 data waves, providing thus another demonstration of developmental generality of the theory, i.e., its invariance across life stages. Second, the findings were similar to those obtained in adolescence in regard to the existence of a problem behavior syndrome, now evident in young adulthood, as well. A variety of analyses showed covariation across frequency of drunkenness, frequency of marijuana use, use of other illicit drugs, general deviant behavior, and cigarette smoking, and also showing that a single underlying factor could account for the observed correlations among those behaviors (Donovan & Jessor, 1985). Third, variation in problem behavior in 1981 was shown to be predictable from psychosocial proneness as far back as 1972/73, i.e., over quite a long developmental period; theoretical precursors in adolescence were able to forecast problem behavior in young adulthood. Fourth, with regard to developmental change in the theoretical predictors and the problem behaviors from adolescence into young adulthood, there is clear evidence of substantial *continuity* in change (Jessor, 1983); stability coefficients between Wave 1 and Wave 6 and between Wave 5 and Wave 6 were highly significant.

Two other important findings about youth development emerged from the Young Adult Follow-Up Study. Despite the observed stability of developmental change, the actual *direction* of change between the adolescent life stage and that of young adulthood "was unmistakably in the direction of greater conventionality" (Jessor et al., 1991, p. 276). This was especially noteworthy given that, for several of the variables, it was an actual reversal of the direction of developmental change observed *within* adolescence when it was toward greater *un*conventionality. Finally, we found that there was no evidence of a "spillover" effect, that is, that involvement in problem behavior in adolescence had compromised young adult outcomes in any other life areas—work, family, health, etc., or that it had "mortgaged the future" of these middle-class youth in any way.

These young adult findings added substantially to our understanding of the implications of the adolescent life stage for later development, They also strengthened our conviction about the developmental usefulness of Problem Behavior Theory in this later stage of the life course.

Part II

Expanding Problem Behavior Theory Beyond Problem Behavior

In carrying out three, large-scale studies of adolescent problem behavior, both cross-sectional and longitudinal, our primary objective had been to innovate a conceptual framework—Problem Behavior Theory—and to establish its usefulness for advancing understanding of the adolescent life stage and the role played by problem behavior in adolescent adaptation and development. The three successive volumes that published the findings from those studies represented a cumulative corpus of work, over several decades, in support of that objective.

But there had been other objectives along the way, as well. A second objective had been to help promote an alternative style of social inquiry: a style that was problem-focused; that could enable strong inferences to be drawn from field or non-experimental studies; that was more comprehensive than what was generally seen in the literature, encompassing both person and environment and engaging a wide range of behaviors; and a style that transcended discipline-focused efforts and reflected what might best be called a *developmental behavioral science* approach (Jessor, 1993), an approach that is inherently interdisciplinary. Related to that objective is the fact that, in 1980, I was appointed director of the Institute of Behavioral Science, a position I held for over two decades, with responsibilities for overseeing a fairly large organized research enterprise with programs on population, the environment, political and economic change, and problem behavior (which I continued to direct, as well). That role required engagement with problem-based, interdisciplinary inquiry across a broad spectrum of the social and behavioral sciences, and it generated an even stronger commitment on my part to promoting developmental behavioral science as an approach to research.

Toward that end, and to celebrate the 25th anniversary of the Institute, I organized in the mid-1980s a 2-year-long series of distinguished lectures on the current and future status of the various social science disciplines, and on such social problems as health, peace, and the environment. Beyond editing the volume *Perspectives on behavioral science: The Colorado lectures* (Jessor, 1991b), I tried in the final chapter, "Behavioral science: An emerging paradigm for social inquiry?" (Jessor, 1991a) to take stock across the lectures of whether a new trans-disciplinary paradigm was, indeed, emerging. Unhappily, I had to conclude that was not the case. That conclusion was not contradicted by a richly rewarding year spent, almost a decade later in 1995–96, at the Center for Advanced Study in the Behavioral Sciences at Stanford. The hold of the disciplinary organization of social-psychological research remains tenacious even today, nearly two decades later, despite the inherent necessity of an inter-or trans-disciplinary perspective when research is problem-based; see invited editorial, "Remarks on the changing nature of inquiry" (Jessor, 2005).

And a third objective was to promote greater reliance on theory in research and measurement. The theoretical or explanatory level of analysis, the level Kurt Lewin (1951), borrowing an analogy from genetics, termed the underlying *genotypic* level, not only provides for logical or systematic explanation, but it also yields greater generality than can be expected from analyses at the descriptive or *phenotypic* levels, which are necessarily parochial. We had already documented the generality of theoretical explanation in the Tri-Ethnic Study in which the theoretical variables showed similar explanatory value across the three ethnic groups despite their varied circumstances and mean-level differences on those variables. Theoretical generality had also been documented across gender and, in the Young Adult Follow-Up Study, across the developmental stage of young adulthood.

Problem Behavior Theory and Adolescent Health. By the early 1980s, Problem Behavior Theory was becoming established and, indeed, beginning to be used by others to guide their own research. Although our third volume, *Beyond adolescence,* had not yet appeared, articles from that study were already being published (e.g., Donovan & Jessor, 1985; Donovan, R. Jessor, & L. Jessor, 1983; Jessor, 1983; Jessor, Donovan, & Costa, 1986; R. Jessor & S.L. Jessor, 1984). With all that as background, the ontogeny of Problem Behavior Theory's development entered a new phase, a phase that was characterized by an expansion of its application into additional domains of adolescent life beyond problem behavior alone.

Perhaps the most salient expansion was engagement of the theory with the domain of *adolescent health.* It had become quite clear to us over the years that many of the adolescent problem behaviors we were preoccupied with, e.g., smoking, alcohol abuse, and early or unprotected sex, could be viewed by those with a public health perspective not as normative transgressions, as we saw them, but as behaviors that compromised health, instead. It was evident, too, that even health-related behaviors that were not also problem behaviors were regulated by social and personal norms just as problem behaviors were, e.g., norms about healthy eating, appropriate exercise, or acceptable body weight, and in that regard it seemed our theory might well be apposite. An invitation by David Hamburg to participate in a conference at the Institute of Medicine served to precipitate an exploration of the applicability of Problem Behavior Theory to the domain of adolescent health, and that led, subsequently, to preparing a chapter, "Adolescent development and behavioral health" (Jessor, 1984) for the volume *Behavioral health: A handbook of health enhancement and disease prevention,* edited by Matarazzo et al. From then on to the present day, concern for the adolescent health domain has threaded its way through our work in research and theory development and across very diverse settings in the United States and across the globe (Costa, Jessor, & Donovan, 1989; Costa, Jessor, Donovan, & Fortenberry, 1995; Donovan, Jessor, & Costa, 1991, 1993; Jessor, 1989; Jessor, Donovan, & Costa, 1990; Jessor, Turbin, & Costa, 1998a, 2010; Turbin, Jessor, & Costa, 2000; Turbin et al., 2006), Indeed, in 2002, I established and became the first director of the Research Program on Health and Society in our Institute of Behavioral Science. Sustaining this engagement with adolescent health, and illuminating its complexity for me, were various opportunities I had to participate in activities that implicated that domain of inquiry. Special mention must be made of service on the Carnegie Council on Adolescent Development for nearly a decade beginning in the mid-80s, which was a richly informative experience. Membership on the National Research Council's Committee on Child Development Research and Public Policy, as well as on its panels, including one on adolescent pregnancy and childbearing and one on high-risk youth, also helped to enlarge my outlook. Involvement in various projects of the World Health Organization, including a cross-national, comparative study of alcohol abuse in Zambia, Mexico, and Scotland, and preparing a presentation, "The health of youth: A behavioral science perspective", for WHO's 1989 Technical Discussions on the Health of Youth, sharpened my awareness of adolescent health issues in the developing world. And serving throughout the 1980s in advisory capacities for various agencies—NIAAA, NIDA, Health and Welfare, Canada—presented the challenge of linking social research on adolescent health to social policy.

A key contribution of Problem Behavior Theory to understanding adolescent health has been to demonstrate the embeddedness of health-related behaviors in a larger explanatory network of psychosocial and behavioral variables. Our research findings established that health behaviors were part of an adolescent's way of being in the world, i.e., part of a *lifestyle.* Health-enhancing behaviors, e.g., healthy diet, regular exercise, adequate sleep, and safety precautions, were shown to inter-relate or co-vary, as was true of problem behaviors; they were also shown to relate inversely to problem behaviors; and they were shown to reflect a general orientation of psychosocial conventionality. Variation in engagement in health-enhancing behavior related not only to proximal variables, such as value on health and attitudes and beliefs about particular health behaviors, variables that directly implicate the health behaviors, but also, and a more novel theoretical finding, to *distal* variables, such as religiosity, as well. These findings added support for the perspective that health behaviors are part of a larger way of being in the world, reflecting an organized, individual-level adolescent lifestyle.

Problem Behavior Theory and the Context of Disadvantage. In addition to its added concern for adolescent health behavior, Problem Behavior Theory also expanded in the 1980s to engage more deeply and directly with adolescent development under circumstances of disadvantage and in contexts of risk, a concern tangentially explored in the early Tri-Ethnic Study. Invited in 1985 by William Bevan to join an advisory group for the MacArthur Foundation's Program on Youth at Risk for Problem Behavior, I was appointed 2 years later as director of a new MacArthur Foundation Research Network on "Successful Adolescent Development among Youth in High Risk Settings," which emerged from the advisory group's deliberations. That began a decade of intense activity by the network members, more than a dozen of the leading scholars on adolescence from psychology, sociology, pediatrics, education, and psychiatry, to try to promote understanding of the process of "making it," i.e., how it is that adolescents growing up under severe conditions of adversity, disadvantage, and even danger nevertheless manage to "succeed": to stay in school and make progress, to avoid heavy engagement in problem behavior, to keep out of trouble with the authorities, to avoid too-early pregnancy or involvement with gangs, etc.

Studies were carried out by interdisciplinary teams of network scholars in inner city poverty neighborhoods in Philadelphia, New York, Chicago, and Denver, as well as in rural Iowa, where farm families had been exposed to the severe economic decline of the 1980s farm crisis. It was a heady experience, enthused with the notion of neighborhood impact on youth development, but also sensitive to other developmental contexts, especially the family and the school, and to individual-level characteristics. An *American Psychologist* article, "Successful adolescent development among youth in high-risk settings" (Jessor, 1993) provided an overview of the network's agenda and approach. Various papers were published from this endeavor, but its main contributions were three converging volumes: *Managing to make it: Urban families and adolescent success* (Furstenberg, Cook, Eccles, & Elder, 1999); *Children of the land: Adversity and success in rural America* (Elder & Conger, 2000); and *Good kids from bad neighborhoods: Successful development in social context* (Elliott et al., 2006). The MacArthur work resulted in significant advances in understanding about adolescent development in high-risk settings, especially in helping to right the balance from a preoccupation with negative outcomes to an emphasis on resources in both person and context, and on positive and successful development. It also revealed, importantly, that there was greater variation *within* neighborhoods than between neighborhoods, and that pure neighborhood effects were, after all, only modest. The MacArthur experience led, in my own work on Problem Behavior Theory, to a related paper, “Risk and protection in successful outcomes among disadvantaged adolescents” (Jessor, Turbin, & Costa, 1998b), which demonstrated the theory’s usefulness in that domain.

Part III

Reformulating Problem Behavior Theory for Explaining Adolescent Risk Behavior: The Current Framework

As the terms “risk” and “protection” in the title of that 1998 article suggest, Problem Behavior Theory had undergone something of a transformation beginning in the early 1990s. The new—and current—formulation extended the theory beyond problem behaviors alone to encompass the broader category of *risk behaviors*, all those behaviors that can compromise adolescent health and successful development. Toward that end, the theory’s predictor or explanatory variables were “translated” into the language of risk factors and protective factors. Adoption of the new formulation was influenced by several things: the accumulated experience of expanding Problem Behavior Theory to apply to the domains of health and disadvantage; discovering that the theory also had reach into hitherto unexplored domains of risk behavior such as “risky driving” (Jessor, 1987b; Jessor et al., 1989); and an awareness of the emergence of a new and relevant subdiscipline of *behavioral* epidemiology, which relied heavily on the concept of “risk factors” and “protective factors,” factors that were congruent with many of our “instigation” and “control” theoretical predictors. The new formulation was designed to make Problem Behavior Theory more readily available to researchers in the health field and more useful for those interested in prevention/intervention, a constituency more familiar with the terminology of “risk” and “protection” than with constructs from our theory such as “problem behavior proneness.”

In what was then for me a pivotal paper, “Risk behavior in adolescence: A psychosocial framework for understanding and action” (Jessor, 1991c), I undertook to create an overarching conceptual framework that could accommodate the variety of theories seeking to account for the broad domain of adolescent risk behavior, including Problem Behavior Theory. It articulated risk factors and protective factors in five different but interrelated domains of “causal” influence: biology/genetics; the social environment; the perceived environment; personality; and behaviors (Fig. 2.3). In requiring specification of both risk and protective factors in each domain, it makes apparent the comprehensiveness and the complexity that a truly exhaustive account of variation in adolescent risk behavior would require. Problem Behavior Theory constitutes one particular derivation from that larger framework.

The incorporation of the concepts of risk behavior, risk factors, and protective factors in that larger framework stimulated some effort to clarify each. First, the concept of “risk behavior,” behaviors that can have health-and life-compromising outcomes, avoids the confusion that has resulted from the pervasive employment of

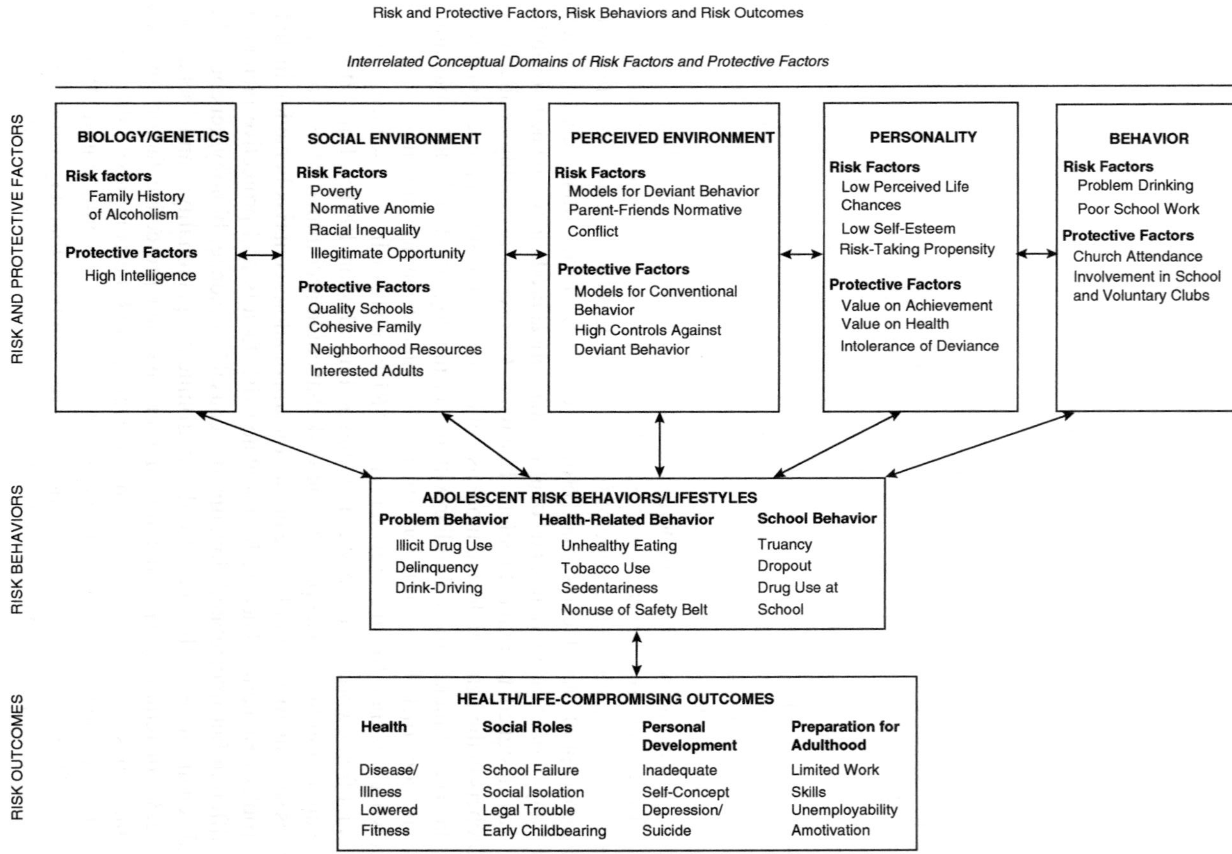

Fig. 2.3 A conceptual framework for adolescent risk behavior (Jessor, 1991c, p. 602)

the term "risk-taking behavior" (with its unsupported corollary that adolescents are, therefore, "risk-takers"). The imputation of risk "taking" is analytically gratuitous when adolescents smoke or drink or have unprotected sex or eat junk food, and use of that term has tended to side-track and even preclude more appropriate explanatory efforts. Whether the deliberate taking of risk is entailed in any of those behaviors needs to be considered as problematic, something to be investigated rather than assumed. The term "risk-taking" has been a source of serious conceptual mischief and should be abandoned—except for those behaviors actually motivated by the conscious thrill of taking the risk involved. In addition, it is also important to recognize that although risk behaviors can compromise health and development, they can also achieve goals the adolescent values, such as a sense of autonomy, or peer approval, or being seen as more mature.

With regard to the concept of "risk factors," it is useful to differentiate the concept into risk factors for the *initiation* of a new risk behavior—its onset—and risk factors for the *intensification of involvement* in or commitment to that risk behavior, once initiated. Since so much of adolescent risk behavior is merely exploratory, the key societal concern has to be with risk factors for intense or committed or chronic involvement with them. With regard to "protective factors", conceptually their *protective* role operates *only when risk is present.* Importantly, in the absence of risk, protective factors play a *promotive* role conceptually, i.e., they provide support for positive, pro-social behavior and development. In addition, protective factors buffer or moderate the impact of exposure to risk factors, i.e., they interact with risk factors to reduce the likelihood of occurrence of risk behavior. It was the recognition of this latter, moderator role of protective factors that led us to shift Problem Behavior Theory from the additive regression model it had always relied on, in regard to instigations and controls, to an interactive model for the risk and protection relationship.

These considerations in mind, we reorganized the theoretical predictors in Problem Behavior Theory into structures of protective factors and risk factors drawn from the "causal" domains of the perceived environment, personality, and behavior. The protective factors that promote positive, pro-social behavior and thereby decrease the likelihood of engaging in risk behavior include: *models* for positive or pro-social behavior; personal and social *controls* against engaging in risk behavior; *social supports* for positive or pro-social behavior; and actual experience with *pro-social or health-enhancing behaviors.* The risk factors that, by contrast, increase the likelihood of occurrence of risk behaviors include: *models* for engaging in risk behavior; *opportunities* for engaging in risk behavior; personal *vulnerability* to engaging in risk behavior; and actual experience with *risk behaviors.* The reformulated Problem Behavior Theory framework used in our research, in one version or another, since the mid-1990s is shown in Fig. 2.4.

The framework illustrates the direct relation of protective factors and risk factors to risk behavior (the direct arrows), as well as the moderator effect of protection on the impact of exposure to risk (the indirect arrow). Both social context and personal variation continue to be represented in the framework. For example, Models Protection refers to perceived models in the adolescent's social environment—family, peers, school, neighborhood—for positive, pro-social, and health-enhancing behav-

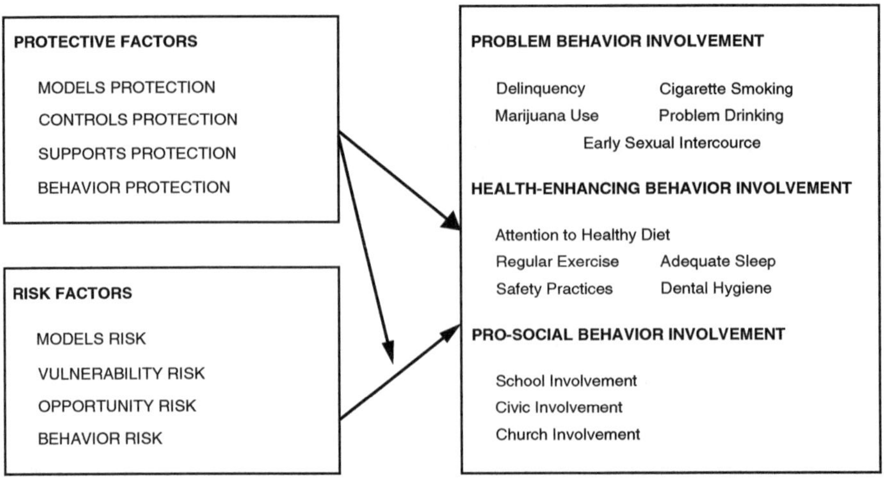

Fig. 2.4 Problem Behavior Theory explanatory model for adolescent risk behavior

ior; Controls Protection refers to informal social controls from peers, family, neighbors, and teachers, as well as personal controls against risk behavior; Vulnerability Risk refers to low self-esteem, low perceived life-chances, and depression at the person-level, all enhancing the likelihood of engaging in risk behavior; etc. The particular variables from Problem Behavior Theory measured in each category of protection and risk can be seen in our various publications (Costa, Jessor, & Turbin, 1999, 2007; Costa et al., 2005; Jessor, Costa, Krueger, & Turbin, 2006; Jessor et al., 1995; Jessor et al., 1998a, b; Jessor et al., 2003; Jessor et al., 2010; Ndugwa et al., 2010; Turbin et al., 2006).

In its latest phase of development, then, the formulation of Problem Behavior Theory has expanded its reach beyond problem behavior to the larger domain of risk behavior in general, and it has brought social-psychological theory to bear in fields that had been largely descriptive, e. g., adolescent health and behavioral epidemiology, by translating its theoretical concepts into risk and protective factors.

Part IV

Problem Behavior Theory in the 21st Century: Establishing Cross-National Generality

The past decade has seen the burgeoning of cross-national applications of Problem Behavior Theory in settings across the globe. The implications that these cross-national efforts have for the generality of findings when research is guided by theory are profound.

Our first systematic application of Problem Behavior Theory in a cross-national study had its origin in an unexpected contact from Professor Qi Dong, a distinguished developmental psychologist at Beijing Normal University, during my 1995–96 year at the Center for Advanced Study in the Behavioral Sciences at Stanford; familiar with my work, he thought it would be mutually beneficial if we could arrange a research collaboration on adolescent development. Intrigued by that possibility, and with funding a couple of years later from the Johann Jacobs Foundation, I organized an international workshop to plan a collaborative, cross-national study of adolescent health and development. The workshop brought together colleagues from Poland and Italy who were already using Problem Behavior Theory in their work, as well as Professor Qi and colleagues from China, and my research group from Colorado. Held in Italy in 1998, the workshop was successful in cementing the U.S.-China collaboration, and an application to the William T. Grant Foundation for a longitudinal research grant, "Adolescent risk behavior and development in China and the U.S.: A cross-national comparative study of risk and protection," was funded in 2000. Our Polish colleagues were ultimately unable to participate, and our Italian colleagues successfully carried out their own Problem Behavior Theory-guided study of Italian youth (Bonino, Cattelino, & Ciairano, 2005).

Most intriguing about the opportunity to test Problem Behavior Theory in The People's Republic of China was how pervasively different from the United States it was as a society and culture: a communist society, a society with a one-child family policy and an extremely low divorce rate, a culture of traditional respect for adults, a relatively lower prevalence of adolescent problem behavior, etc. Successful application of the theory in such a different societal context would provide compelling evidence of its generality. To insure that societal contrast, the study also included a city, Zhengzhou, in central China, which was less exposed than Beijing to Western influence. A comparative, school-based, longitudinal study of adolescent risk behavior was carried out in parallel in the two cities in China and in the city of Denver in the United States. Its findings have been reported in several U.S. publications (Costa et al., 2005; Jessor et al., 2003; Jessor et al., 2010; Turbin et al., 2006), as well as in publications in China.

Whether the analytic focus was on adolescent problem behavior, on pro-social behavior, or on health-enhancing behavior, there was strong support for the cross-national generality of the protection-risk explanatory model of Problem Behavior Theory. A substantial account of variation in risk behavior was provided by the same protective and risk factors in both countries, and for both genders, despite the large societal and cultural differences and despite differences in prevalence of the behaviors and in mean levels on the theoretical predictors. Of further importance, and as theoretically expected, protection was shown also to moderate the impact of exposure to risk in both countries. Just one important finding from this research: When the criterion was problem behavior, Controls Protection and Models Risk were the main predictors in both countries, but when the criterion was positive, that is, either pro-social or health-enhancing behavior, the important predictors shifted to Models Protection, Support Protection, and Vulnerability Risk, an entirely different pattern. Such findings attest to the value of differentiating both risk and protection and the necessity of considering such differentiation in prevention/intervention efforts.

Later, in collaboration with the African Population and Health Research Center in Nairobi, another cross-national study, with adolescents in the slums that surround the city, constituted the first application of Problem Behavior Theory in sub-Saharan Africa. In this contrasting setting from the U.S. contexts in which the theory had been developed, measures of the theory's psychosocial protective and risk factor variables again provided a substantial account of variation in adolescent problem behavior, and protection was again shown to moderate the impact of exposure to risk (Kabiru, Beguy, Ndugwa, Zulu, & Jessor, 2012; Ndugwa et al., 2010).

Our studies in The People's Republic of China and in Kenya provided persuasive support for the cross-national applicability of Problem Behavior Theory. But the establishment of its generality by other, independent investigators makes that support even more convincing, and considerable literature has accumulated in recent years in that very regard. For example, Vazsonyi and colleagues (2008, 2010) report on their application of Problem Behavior Theory in cross-national studies, one using large, national probability samples of adolescents in Switzerland and The Republic of Georgia, and the other using convenience school samples from Hungary, the Netherlands, Slovenia, Spain, Switzerland, Taiwan, Turkey, and the United States. The former study supported the concept of a "problem behavior syndrome" in both societies, and confirmed that Problem Behavior Theory "has applicability across developmental contexts or societies" (2008, p. 562). The latter study concluded that: "The evidence appears to support great similarities in the relationships between risk and protective factors and the PBS [problem behavior syndrome] across the eight developmental contexts" (2010, p. 7). In another cross-national study, of early adolescent sexual initiation in Finland, Scotland, France, Poland, and the United States, Madkour et al. used Problem Behavior Theory as their framework; they conclude that "the fit of early adolescent sexual initiation within a PBT [Problem Behavior Theory] framework holds for multiple post-industrial national settings" (Madkour, Farhat, Halpern, Godeau, & Gabhainn, 2010, p. 397). By now, Problem Behavior Theory has been employed successfully in numerous other countries as well, ranging from Italy and the Netherlands (Ciairano, Kliewer, & Rabaglietti, 2009) to Ethiopia (Astatke, Black, & Serpell, 2000) to Iran (Aguilar-Vafaie, Roshani, Hassanabadi, Masoudian, & Afruz, 2011).

These consistent findings about the applicability of a theory devised and established in the United States to such widely differing societal and cultural contexts often startle or surprise, but as I indicated in an invited editorial, "Description versus explanation in cross-national research on adolescence," for the *Journal of Adolescent Health* when it published the 2008 Vazsonyi et al. paper, such generality is to be expected *at the theoretical level* (Jessor, 2008). Since a theory specifies underlying relations among variables, those relations should obtain in any context in which the theory can be applied—that is the nature of *explanatory* research. In considering the theoretical concept of "Support Protection," for example, its source may come from a single mother in a U.S. family or from an extended-kin group in China or from peers in the slums of Nairobi, but the theoretical relation of support protection to risk behavior should be the same in all three settings. It is this genotypic, explanatory role of theory that yields generality across phenotypic or descriptive differences in populations and contexts. Our studies have thus far supported the generality of the theory across ethnic groups, across gender, across life stages, across historically different U.S. cohorts (Donovan et al., 1999), and across widely diverse societies.

Concluding Reflections

The Problem Behavior Theory that has evolved from this half-century of cumulative work has, it is hoped, contributed to knowledge and understanding about adolescence along the way. As was true of the prior versions, its current protection/risk formulation is predicated on fundamental social-psychological processes that, underlie behavior and shape the course of development both positively and negatively: social *models*; social and personal *controls;* social *supports;* contextual *opportunity;* personal *vulnerability*; and past engagement in risk, health, and pro-social *behaviors.* Although its early focus was on problem behavior, its applications to pro-social domains, including health enhancing behavior, have been equally illuminating. This should not really be surprising; as the criminologist, Albert Cohen, pointed out: "A theory of deviant behavior not only must account for the occurrence of deviant behavior; it must also account for its failure to occur, or conformity" (1959, p. 463). This broader scope of Problem Behavior Theory is the legacy of a long-term, developmental behavioral science approach to inquiry.

That approach insists on the joint consideration of social environment and individual-level determinants of action. The distinguished personality psychologist, Henry Murray, asserted about the time that our work began that "no theoretical system constructed on the psychological level will be adequate until it has been embraced by and intermeshed with a cultural-sociological system" (1959, p. 20). From our early engagement with the socio-cultural system in the Tri-Ethnic Study to our recent concern for articulating risk and protective factors in the social contexts of daily adolescent life, we have sought to embrace the social environment in an interdisciplinary formulation for understanding adolescent behavior and development. And in documenting the unique variance added by the social environment measures to accounts based only on individual-level variables (Costa et al., 2005; Turbin et al., 2006), our findings have exemplified interdisciplinary research.

Complementing this engagement with the social environment has been our parallel interest in understanding the phenomenal world of the adolescent. From the very outset, the Tri-Ethnic Study was informed by extensive ethnographic explorations in the community; and in the three MacArthur volumes, ethnographic findings became an essential component of those studies. Indeed, the necessity to join qualitative with quantitative inquiry in order to achieve a deeper understanding of the impact of disadvantage on adolescent development quickly became apparent in the network, and toward that end, we organized a symposium on qualitative research that eventuated in an illuminating volume, *Ethnography and human development: Context and meaning in social inquiry* (Jessor, 1996; Jessor, Colby, & Shweder, 1996). It has been dismaying to continue to confront the intractable opposition of post-modernism in sociology and anthropology to quantitative work and the equally obstinate perspective of some quantitative social scientists about qualitative research; the volume bravely sought to overcome that polarity. We should be long past awarding honorific status to particular methods; methods serve as handmaidens to theory and problems.

As I look back now over more than five decades of research on adolescence, I'm most aware of how much remains to be accomplished. As successful as Problem Behavior Theory may have been—its social-psychological variables accounting in some cases for as much as half the variance in risk behavior—it is sobering to realize that fully half the variance remains unexplained; therein lies the challenge for the developmental science of adolescence in future years. One promising avenue to pursue in response to that challenge is engaging additional disciplines in the explanatory scheme. In this regard, it has been salutary to see the burgeoning attention to neuroscience and genetics in contemporary adolescent research. A caveat about following that course is in order, however; findings from those disciplines are too often considered as somehow more fundamental and more causal than findings at the social-psychological level, a kind of reductionist fallacy that can seriously skew scientific progress. Recent explanations of risk behavior based on the so-called "immature adolescent brain" or references to "addictive" behavior as a "brain disease"—especially in the absence of evidence about linking mechanisms—are two examples. In a long-ago article, "The problem of reductionism in psychology" (Jessor, 1958), I tried to argue against this tendency; more recently, Miller (2010) has addressed the issue in greater detail.

Another promising direction to pursue is gaining a deeper understanding of the social context of adolescent life. It is now clear to everyone that the standard demographic attributes—the so-called "social addresses"—are too distal to be helpful. Developing a more sensitive and differentiated theoretical language to describe the contexts of adolescent daily life, one that could better capture the learnings and rewards and opportunities and sanctions that exist in those settings, should yield a stronger grasp on the role of the social environment than we have yet achieved. Finally, probing more deeply the adolescent's phenomenology, getting at the quiddities of adolescent subjectivity, could certainly enrich understanding.

There is, of course, a sense of satisfaction in looking back at the contribution that Problem Behavior Theory has made to a developmental science of adolescence; at the same time, there is a continuing sense of excitement over addressing the challenges that remain for that still-emerging science.

> Behind all scientific studies there is not only the drive to understand but the compulsion to persuade.
>
> William Bevan

Acknowledgments I am indebted to my students and colleagues who have, over the years, contributed immensely to the work described in this chapter. Many are named in the citations and references, but to all of them I am grateful for their ideas and their efforts. Three colleagues, Frances M. Costa, John E. Donovan, and Mark S. Turbin, deserve special mention and warm appreciation for their involvement in our most recent research.

References

Aguilar-Vafaie, M. E., Roshani, M., Hassanabadi, H., Masoudian, Z., & Afruz, G. A. (2011). Risk and protective factors for residential foster care adolescents. *Children and Youth. Services Review, 33*, 1–15.

Astatke, H., Black, M. M., & Serpell, R. (2000). Use of Jessor's theoretical framework of adolescent risk behavior in Ethiopia: Implications for HIV/AIDS prevention. *Northeast African Studies, 7*, 63–68.

Blau, P. M., Gustad, J. W., Jessor, R., Parnes, H. S., & Wilcock, R. C. (1956). Occupational choice: A conceptual framework. *Industrial & Labor Relations Review, 9*(4), 531–543.

Bonino, S., Cattelino, E., & Ciairano, S. (2005). *Adolescents and risk: Behaviors, functions, and protective factors*. New York: Springer.

Ciairano, S., Kliewer, W., & Rabaglietti, E. (2009). Adolescent risk behavior in Italy and the Netherlands: A cross-national study of psychosocial protective factors. *European Psychologist, 14*, 180–192.

Cloward, R. A., & Ohlin, L. E. (1960). *Delinquency and opportunity: A theory of delinquent gangs*. New York: Free Press.

Cohen, A. K. (1959). The study of social disorganization and deviant behavior. In R. K. Merton, L. Broom, & L. S. Cottrell Jr. (Eds.), *Sociology today: Problems and prospects* (pp. 461–484). New York: Basic Books.

Costa, F. (2008). *Problem behavior theory: A brief overview*. Available at: www.colorado.edu/ibs/Jessor/pb_theory.html.

Costa, F. M., Jessor, R., & Donovan, J. E. (1989). Value on health and adolescent conventionality: A construct validation of a new measure in Problem Behavior Theory. *Journal of Applied Social Psychology, 19*(10), 841–861.

Costa, F. M., Jessor, R., Donovan, J. E., & Fortenberry, J. D. (1995). Early initiation of sexual intercourse: The influence of psychosocial unconventionality. *Journal of Research on Adolescence, 5*(1), 93–121.

Costa, F. M., Jessor, R., & Turbin, M. S. (1999). Transition into adolescent problem drinking: The role of psychosocial risk and protective factors. *Journal of Studies on Alcohol, 60*(4), 480–490.

Costa, F. M., Jessor, R., & Turbin, M. S. (2007). College student involvement in cigarette smoking: The role of psychosocial and behavioral protection and risk. *Nicotine & Tobacco Research, 9*(2), 213–224.

Costa, F. M., Jessor, R., Turbin, M. S., Dong, Q., Zhang, H., & Wang, C. (2005). The role of social contexts in adolescence: Context protection and context risk in the U.S. and China. *Applied Developmental Science, 9*, 67–85.

Cronbach, L. J., & Meehl, P. E. (1955). Construct validity in psychological tests. *Psychological Bulletin, 52*(4), 281–302.

Donovan, J. E. (2005). Problem behavior theory. In C. B. Fisher & R. M. Lerner (Eds.), *Encyclopedia of applied developmental science* (Vol. 2, pp. 872–877). Thousand Oaks, CA: Erudite.

Donovan, J. E., & Jessor, R. (1978). Adolescent problem drinking: Psychosocial correlates in a national sample study. *Journal of Studies on Alcohol, 39*(9), 1506–1524.

Donovan, J. E., & Jessor, R. (1985). Structure of problem behavior in adolescence and young adulthood. *Journal of Consulting and Clinical Psychology, 53*(6), 890–904.

Donovan, J. E., Jessor, R., & Costa, F. M. (1991). Adolescent health behavior and conventionality-unconventionality: An extension of Problem Behavior Theory. *Health Psychology, 10*(1), 52–61.

Donovan, J. E., Jessor, R., & Costa, F. M. (1993). Structure of health-enhancing behavior in adolescence: A latent-variable approach. *Journal of Health and Social Behavior, 34*(4), 346–362.

Donovan, J. E., Jessor, R., & Costa, F. M. (1999). Adolescent problem drinking: Stability of psychosocial and behavioral correlates across a generation. *Journal of Studies on Alcohol, 60*(3), 352–361.

Donovan, J. E., Jessor, R., & Jessor, L. (1983). Problem drinking in adolescence and young adulthood: A follow-up study. *Journal of Studies on Alcohol, 44*(1), 109–137.

Elder, G. H., & Conger, R. D. (2000). *Children of the land: Adversity and success in rural America*. Chicago: University of Chicago Press.
Elliott, D. S., Menard, S., Rankin, B., Elliott, A., Wilson, W. J., & Huizinga, D. (2006). *Good kids from bad neighborhoods: Successful development in social context*. New York: Cambridge University Press.
Furstenberg, F. F., Jr., Cook, T. D., Eccles, J., & Eider, G. H. (1999). *"Managing to make it": Urban families and adolescent success*. Chicago: University of Chicago Press.
Gruber, H. E., Hammond, K. R., & Jessor, R. (Eds.). (1957). *Contemporary approaches to cognition*. Cambridge: Harvard University Press.
Hull, C. L. (1943). *Principles of behavior: An introduction to behavior theory*. New York: D. Appleton-Century Company.
Jessor, R. (1956). Phenomenological personality theories and the data language of psychology. *Psychological Review, 63*(3), 173–180.
Jessor, R. (1958). The problem of reductionism in psychology. *Psychological Review, 65*(3), 170–178.
Jessor, R. (1976). Predicting time of onset of marijuana use: A developmental study of high school youth. *Journal of Consulting and Clinical Psychology, 44*(1), 125–134.
Jessor, R. (1983). The stability of change: Psychosocial development from adolescence to young adulthood. In D. Magnusson & V. L. Allen (Eds.), *Human development: An interactional perspective* (pp. 321–341). New York: Academic Press.
Jessor, R. (1984). Adolescent development and behavioral health. In J. D. Matarazzo, S. M. Weiss, J. A. Herd, & N. E. Miller (Eds.), *Behavioral health: A handbook of health enhancement and disease prevention* (pp. 69–90). New York: Wiley.
Jessor, R. (1987a). Problem behavior theory, psychosocial development, and adolescent problem drinking. *British Journal of Addiction, 82*(4), 331–342.
Jessor, R. (1987b). Risky driving and adolescent problem behavior: Theoretical and empirical linkage. *Alcohol, Drugs, and Driving, 3*, 1–11.
Jessor, R. (1991a). Behavioral science: An emerging paradigm for social inquiry? In R. Jessor (Ed.), *Perspectives on behavioral science: The Colorado lectures* (pp. 309–316). Boulder, CO: Westview Press.
Jessor, R. (Ed.). (1991b). *Perspectives on behavioral science: The Colorado lectures*. Boulder, CO: Westview Press.
Jessor, R. (1991c). Risk behavior in adolescence: A psychosocial framework for understanding and action. *Journal of Adolescent Health, 12*(8), 597–605.
Jessor, R. (1993). Successful adolescent development among youth in high-risk settings. *American Psychologist, 48*(2), 117–126.
Jessor, R. (1996). Ethnographic methods in contemporary perspective. In R. Jessor, A. Colby, & R. A. Shweder (Eds.), *Ethnography and human development: Context and meaning in social inquiry* (pp. 3–14). Chicago: University of Chicago Press.
Jessor, R. (2005). Remarks on the changing nature of inquiry. *Journal of Adolescent Health, 37*(1), 9–10.
Jessor, R. (2008). Description versus explanation in cross-national research on adolescence. *Journal of Adolescent Health, 43*(6), 527–528.
Jessor, R., Chase, J. A., & Donovan, J. E. (1980). Psychosocial correlates of marijuana use and problem drinking in a national sample of adolescents. *American Journal of Public Health, 70*(6), 604–613.
Jessor, R., Colby, A., & Shweder, R. A. (Eds.). (1996). *Ethnography and human development: Context and meaning in social inquiry*. Chicago: University of Chicago Press.
Jessor, R., Costa, F., Jessor, S. L., & Donovan, J. E. (1983). Time of first intercourse: A prospective study. *Journal of Personality and Social Psychology, 44*, 608–626.
Jessor, R., Costa, F. M., Krueger, P. M., & Turbin, M. S. (2006). A developmental study of heavy episodic drinking among college students: The role of psychosocial and behavioral protective and risk factors. *Journal of Studies on Alcohol, 67*(1), 86–94.
Jessor, R., Donovan, J. E., & Costa, F. (1986). Psychosocial correlates of marijuana use in adolescence and young adulthood: The past as prologue. *Alcohol, Drugs, and Driving, 2*, 31–49.

Jessor, R., Donovan, J. E., & Costa, F. (1989). Problem drinking and risky driving among youth: A psychosocial approach to a lifestyle pattern, in *Proceedings, International Conference on High Alcohol Consumers and Traffic* (pp. 137-152). Paris: INRETS.

Jessor, R., Donovan, J. E., & Costa, F. (1990). Personality, perceived life chances, and adolescent health behavior: An application of Problem Behavior Theory. In K. Hurrelmann & F. Lösel (Eds.), *Health hazards in adolescence* (pp. 25–41). Hawthorne, NY: Aldine/De Gruyter.

Jessor, R., Donovan, J. E., & Costa, F. M. (1991). *Beyond adolescence: Problem behavior and young adult development*. New York: Cambridge University Press.

Jessor, R., Graves, T. D., Hanson, R. C., & Jessor, S. L. (1968). *Society, personality, and deviant behavior: A study of a tri-ethnic community*. New York: Holt, Rinehart and Winston.

Jessor, R., & Hammond, K. R. (1957). Construct validity and the Taylor Anxiety Scale. *Psychological Bulletin, 54*(3), 161–170.

Jessor, R., & Jessor, S. L. (1973). The perceived environment in behavioral science: Some conceptual issues and some illustrative data. *American Behavioral Scientist, 16*(6), 801–828.

Jessor, R., & Jessor, S. L. (1975a). Adolescent development and the onset of drinking: A longitudinal study. *Journal of Studies on Alcohol, 36*(1), 27–51.

Jessor, R., & Jessor, S. L. (1977). *Problem behavior and psychosocial development: A longitudinal study of youth*. New York: Academic Press.

Jessor, R., & Jessor, S. L. (1984). Adolescence to young adulthood: A twelve-year prospective study of problem behavior and psychosocial development. In S. A. Mednick, M. Harway, & K. M. Finello (Eds.), *Handbook of longitudinal research* (Teenage and adult cohorts, Vol. 2, pp. 34–61). New York: Praeger.

Jessor, R., Jessor, S. L., & Collins, M. I. (1972). On becoming a drinker: Social-psychological aspects of an adolescent transition. In F. A. Seixas (Ed.), *Nature and nurture in alcoholism* (pp. 199–213). New York: Annals of the New York Academy of Sciences.

Jessor, R., Turbin, M. S., & Costa, F. M. (1998a). Protective factors in adolescent health behavior. *Journal of Personality and Social Psychology, 75*(3), 788–800.

Jessor, R., Turbin, M. S., & Costa, F. M. (1998b). Risk and protection in successful outcomes among disadvantaged adolescents. *Applied Developmental Science, 2*, 194–208.

Jessor, R., Turbin, M. S., & Costa, F. M. (2010). Predicting developmental change in healthy eating and regular exercise among adolescents in China and the United States: The role of psychosocial and behavioral protection and risk. *Journal of Research on Adolescence, 20*(3), 707–725.

Jessor, R., Turbin, M. S., Costa, F. M., Dong, Q., Zhang, H. C., & Wang, C. H. (2003). Adolescent problem behavior in China and the United States: A cross-national study of psychosocial protective factors. *Journal of Research on Adolescence, 13*(3), 329–360.

Jessor, R., Van Den Bos, J., Vanderryn, J., Costa, F. M., & Turbin, M. S. (1995). Protective factors in adolescent problem behavior: Moderator effects and developmental change. *Developmental Psychology, 31*(6), 923–933.

Jessor, R., Young, H. B., Young, E. B., & Tesi, G. (1970). Perceived opportunity, alienation, and drinking behavior among Italian and American youth. *Journal of Personality and Social Psychology, 15*(3), 215–222.

Jessor, S. L., & Jessor, R. (1975b). Transition from virginity to nonvirginity among youth: A social-psychological study over time. *Developmental Psychology, 11*(4), 473–484.

Kabiru, C. W., Beguy, D., Ndugwa, R. P., Zulu, E. M., & Jessor, R. (2012). "Making it": Understanding adolescent resilience in two informal settlements (slums) in Nairobi. *Kenya, Child and Youth Services, 33*, 12–32.

Lewin, K. (1935). *A dynamic theory of personality: Selected papers*. New York: McGraw-Hill.

Lewin, K. (1951). *Field theory in social science: Selected theoretical papers*. New York: Harper & Row.

Madkour, A. S., Farhat, T., Halpern, C. T., Godeau, E., & Gabhainn, S. N. (2010). Early adolescent sexual initiation as a problem behavior: A comparative study of five nations. *Journal of Adolescent Health, 47*(4), 389–398.

Merton, R. K. (1957). *Social theory and social structure* (Rev. and enl.th ed.). New York: Free Press.

Miller, G. A. (2010). Mistreating psychology in the decades of the brain. *Perspectives on Psychological Science, 5*(6), 716–743.

Monahan, K. C., & Hawkins, J. D. (2012). Covariance of problem behaviors in adolescence. Paper presented at IOM Committee on the Science of Adolescence Workshop. Washington, DC.

Murray, H. A. (1959). Preparations for the scaffold of a comprehensive system. In S. Koch (Ed.), *Psychology: A study of a science* (Vol. 3, pp. 7–54). New York: McGraw-Hill.

Ndugwa, R. P., Kabiru, C. W., Cleland, J., Beguy, D., Egondi, T., Zulu, E. M., et al. (2010). Adolescent problem behavior in Nairobi's informal settlements: Applying Problem Behavior Theory in sub-Saharan Africa. *Journal of Urban Health, 88*(Suppl. 2), 298–317.

Parsons, T. (1937). *The structure of social action: A study in social theory with special reference to a group of recent European writers*. New York: McGraw-Hill.

Rachal, J. V., Williams, J. R., & Brehm, M. L. (1975). *A national study of adolescent drinking behavior, attitudes, and correlates. (Rep. No. PB-246-002; NIAAA/NCALI-75/27)*. Springfield, VA: National Technical Information Service.

Rogers, C. R. (1959). A theory of therapy, personality, and interpersonal relationships as developed in the client-centered framework. In S. Koch (Ed.), *Psychology: A study of a science* (Vol. 3, pp. 184–256). New York: McGraw-Hill.

Rotter, J. B. (1954). *Social learning and clinical psychology*. Englewood Cliffs, NJ: Prentice-Hall.

Skinner, B. F. (1938). *The behavior of organisms: An experimental analysis*. New York: D. Appleton-Century Company.

Thomas, W. I. (1928). *The child in America: Behavior problems and programs*. New York: Alfred A. Knopf.

Turbin, M. S., Jessor, R., & Costa, F. M. (2000). Adolescent cigarette smoking: Health-related behavior or normative transgression? *Prevention Science, 1*, 115–124.

Turbin, M. S., Jessor, R., Costa, F. M., Dong, Q., Zhang, H. C., & Wang, C. H. (2006). Protective and risk factors in health-enhancing behavior among adolescents in China and the United States: Does social context matter? *Health Psychology, 25*(4), 445–454.

Vazsonyi, A. T., Chen, P., Jenkins, D. D., Burcu, E., Torrente, G., & Sheu, C.-J. (2010). Jessor's problem behavior theory: Cross-national evidence from Hungary, the Netherlands, Slovenia, Spain, Switzerland, Taiwan, Turkey, and the United States. *Developmental Psychology, 46*(6), 1779–1791.

Vazsonyi, A. T., Chen, P., Young, M., Jenkins, D., Browder, S., Kahumoku, E., et al. (2008). A test of Jessor's problem behavior theory in a Eurasian and a Western European developmental context. *Journal of Adolescent Health, 43*(6), 555–564.

Chapter 3
Problem Behavior Theory: Initial Formulation for the Tri-Ethnic Community Study

Richard Jessor, Theodore D. Graves, Robert C. Hanson, and Shirley L. Jessor

In this book (Jessor, Graves, Hanson, & Jessor, 1968) we have sought to inform the reader about what we have done and how we went about our work. We described the initial problem which we assumed as the explanatory objective, the concepts we used in a theoretical formulation, the stance we took with respect to field research, the measures devised and the studies in which they were employed, and, finally, the results that were obtained. A review of these various aspects should be useful at this point; discussion of problems and issues raised by the research and some of its limitations and implications will follow.

A Brief Overview

The research began with the task of accounting for the differential rates of occurrence of problem behavior, especially heavy alcohol use, among three ethnic groups in a small rural community in southwestern Colorado. Although members of the community were ready with their own "explanations," and although there were several obvious vantage points from which an investigation might begin, it seemed clear that the situation provided a natural laboratory in which a general theory of

Reprinted with permission from:
Jessor, R., Graves, T. D., Hanson, R. C., & Jessor, S. L. (1968). Chapter 13: "Overview and appraisal of theory and findings." In R. Jessor, T. D. Graves, R. C. Hanson & S. L. Jessor, *Society, personality, and deviant behavior: A study of a tri-ethnic community* (pp. 407–421). New York: Holt, Rinehart and Winston.

T.D. Graves • R.C. Hanson • S.L. Jessor
(deceased)

R. Jessor (✉)
Institute of Behavioral Science, University of Colorado at Boulder, Boulder, CO 80309, USA
e-mail: jessor@Colorado.edu

R. Jessor, *The Origins and Development of Problem Behavior Theory*,
Advancing Responsible Adolescent Development,
DOI 10.1007/978-3-319-40886-6_3

deviance-conformity might be developed and put to test. The accomplishment of such an objective required a conceptual analysis of the behavior involved and of the factors, in both the person and the situation, which might be important influences upon it.

Our first concern was to recognize the essential continuity between deviance and conformity and to assume that an explanation focused at either pole must have implications for the other. What this implied was that deviant behavior, like any other, was best treated as learned, purposive, goal oriented, in short, as adaptive action requiring no special principles to account for its occurrence beyond those required for social behavior in general. The central issue became that of explaining not deviance per se but the occurrence of deviant rather than some other, that is, conforming, behavior. Stated otherwise, the problem was to account for selection or choice among possible adaptive alternatives. In this light, the selection of deviant behavioral adaptations, despite the ultimate possibility of negative sanctions, appeared to be more likely when other alternatives had come to be seen by the actor as promising him little in the way of success. The view that it would be useful to interpret deviance as reflecting, at least in part, the failure of conformity was adopted.

Our second concern was to recognize the complexity inherent in the concept of deviance. One source of complexity stems from the diversity of behavior which the concept subsumes. Any number of actions, all significantly departing from normative prescription, can be learned as alternative adaptations when conforming behavior fails to secure personal goals. The recognition of this source of complexity suggested the need to go beyond a concern with heavy alcohol use alone to include other adaptations which might be functionally equivalent. A test of a theory of deviant behavior seemed to us to require an assessment of the class of deviant alternatives rather than a focus upon any particular one. A second source of complexity is that which inheres in all social behavior: the fact that deviance and conformity represent the outcome of multiple influences and determinants in both the person and his situation.

These views about deviant behavior directed our analysis of both personality and the sociocultural environment, an analysis demanding multiple determinants likely to reflect the failure of conformity and the availability of deviant alternatives. For the major personality formulations, we drew upon Rotter's social learning theory (1954); for the sociocultural concepts, we borrowed from Merton (1957), and Cloward and Ohlin (1961). Complementary, analogous conceptualizations of the person and of the environment, systematically coordinated to each other and to deviance, were consequently developed.

The sociocultural environment was articulated as a system made up of three major structures: the opportunity structure, the normative structure, and the social control structure. Location in the opportunity structure was construed as a source of pressure toward the adoption of illegitimate means, with low access to opportunity implying a relatively high degree of pressure. Locations in both the normative structure and the social control structure were defined as sources of controls against the adoption of illegitimate means, with high anomie in the normative structure and high access to illegitimate means in the social control structure implying a low degree of control. Deviance as a sociocultural outcome was, therefore, considered to be the resultant of sociocultural pressure and controls, neither factor alone yielding a sufficient explanation.

The same conceptual approach was applied to the person. Personality was construed as a system made up of three structures parallel to those constituting the sociocultural system: a perceived opportunity structure, providing a source of pressure toward deviance, and a personal belief structure and a personal control structure, both representing personal controls against engaging in deviance. The resultant of personal pressure and control was seen to determine, now at the personality level, the likelihood of deviant behavior, neither factor alone being sufficient.

Although these two conceptual systems, sociocultural and personality constitute separate theories of deviance, their formal similarity and parallel concepts enabled their assimilation into a single, interdisciplinary, explanatory scheme. This was our basic objective: to construct a field theory of deviant behavior in which the interaction of sociocultural and personality determinants could be dealt with systematically.

To make the field theory a more convincing synthesis, it seemed important to consider how the sociocultural environment comes, over time, to influence the development of personality. To this end, socialization was construed as a system lying at the interface between society and the person. It also was articulated into three structures, ones likely to reflect the sociocultural system and, at the same time, to be relevant to the personality system. The structures of the socialization system, analogues of the structures in the other two systems, were the parental reward structure, the parental belief structure, and the parental control structure.

A test of the adequacy of the explanatory formulation was seen to rest on its ability to yield, simultaneously, an account of differences between ethnic groups in rates of occurrence of deviance and an account of individual differences within the community and within ethnic groups in the occurrence-nonoccurrence of deviance. The logic of the approach was that the same factors used to explain individual behavior could be applied to explaining differences between groups of individuals, in our case, ethnic groups. The implication of this logic for the meaning of the concept of ethnic status will be elaborated later on.

Second to, and influenced by, our concern for theory was our commitment to developing a research methodology appropriate to the testing of theory in field studies. Although field studies are usually seen as part of the context of exploration and discovery, it was our view that they are also appropriate to the context of justification. To fulfill this latter role, to be relevant to the testing of propositions, field studies require design in which consistent efforts to minimize inferential ambiguity are made. For us this meant, beyond the usual concern for standardization and reliable measurement, the logical derivation of measuring procedures from concepts, the development of multiple measures of concepts, and the use of multiple, converging studies, each independent of the others but converging upon the validity of the over-all social-psychological framework. To the extent that such a methodological orientation could be successfully implemented, to that extent, it seemed to us, could theory-testing be compelling in field research.

Three separate and independent studies were carried out in the community. The first of these was a community survey study in which data were collected by individual interview from a random sample of adults between the ages of twenty and sixty-five, stratified by sex and ethnic group. The interview included measures of the sociocultural system, the personality system, and the behavior system, that is, deviance-conformity and alcohol use. Information on the latter was supplemented by an exhaustive search of relevant court records but, in the main, this study provided a self-contained test of the theory based upon self-report interview data. The second study focused upon a younger age group in the community, the students in the local high school. It involved a wide range of procedures, including self-report group questionnaires, interviews, sociometrics, behavior tests, teacher ratings, and school records. Yielding sociocultural, personality, and behavior measures, it enabled a second, independent test of the over-all framework.

The third study dealt with socialization and was an attempt to study the linkage between the sociocultural system, on the one hand, and the personality and behavior systems, on the other. In the socialization study, data were collected by individual interview from the mothers of the students in the high school, and measures based upon these data were used to predict the personality and behavior measures independently obtained from their children in the high school.

All three studies provided some degree of support for the theory guiding the research, and the convergence of the findings from the separate studies constitutes a strong basis for inference. Among the ethnic groups, the Anglos were shown to occupy the most favorable position in the opportunity structure: They have the greatest objective access to valued goals by legitimate means and are, consequently, under the least pressure to adopt alternative, often illegitimate, means. With respect to the normative structure, they were also shown to occupy the most theoretically favorable position: they have the greatest degree of consensus around group norms, that is, the least anomie, and are subject, therefore, to the greatest normative control against the adoption of illegitimate means. Finally, with respect to the social control structure, their position is also the most favorable: they have least access to illegitimate means and are, therefore, subject to the strongest social controls. Taken together, the findings show the Anglos to occupy the point of intersection in sociocultural "space" which should be theoretically least conducive to deviance, the point, relative to the other two ethnic groups, at which pressures toward deviance are lowest and controls against deviance are highest. These findings are consistent with the data showing that the Anglos, among the three ethnic groups, make the least contribution to deviance rates in the community.

Considering the other two ethnic groups, the Spanish and the Indians, the findings are more complex and make clear the utility of a theory which deals simultaneously with both pressures and controls. In terms of pressures toward deviance, the Indians actually have a somewhat more favorable position in the opportunity structure than the Spanish, at least when access to opportunity is defined exclusively in terms of socioeconomic status. With respect to controls, however, the Spanish clearly occupy the theoretically more favorable position. The measure of normative controls suggests that anomie is more pervasive and generalized among the Indians than among the Spanish; and with respect to social controls, the picture is sharpest, the Spanish having least exposure to deviant role models and being mapped into solidary sanctioning networks such as the Catholic Church, the family, and informal groups significantly more than are the Indians. Despite equal or even greater pressures toward deviance, the Spanish are subject to the operation of much stronger and more consistent controls than the Indians. These findings are consonant with the data showing the Indians to contribute most to the deviance rates in the community, with the Spanish intermediate between them and the Anglos. The intermediate position of the Spanish rates is actually much closer to that of the Anglos than it is to that of the Indians, suggesting the possibly more important role played by social controls, relative to pressures, in influencing the occurrence of deviance.

The findings just described support the sociocultural aspect of the theory in dealing with ethnic group differences in deviant behavior. The results bearing on the personality aspect of the theory are also supportive. The Anglos have the greatest *perception* of opportunity, that is, the highest expectations of achieving goals, or the least personal disjunctions. They are also least alienated with respect to the personal belief structure, and they have the strongest personal controls. The trend with respect to the two minority groups is for the Indians to hold the more deviance-prone position on the personality measures compared to the Spanish, although the relative position of the two groups is not clearly established on all of the measures. With respect to personal control measures, however, as was the case with social controls, the Spanish, despite their low position in the economic opportunity structure, are closer to the Anglos than they are to the Indians.

The support provided for the over-all social-psychological framework by the outcome just described gains reinforcement from the fact that it emerges from two independent studies in the community, one dealing with adults and the other with adolescents of high school age. These two studies, using different age groups, different measures, and different settings, yet generating congruent empirical data, yield the kind of convergence toward which the methodological planning was oriented. Further convergence stems from the socialization study. Ethnic group differences in parental reward structure, parental belief structure, and parental control structure measures follow from the sociocultural position of the family and accord with the personality and behavior measures of the high school children.

Showing that ethnic group differences in deviance rates were consonant with the relative positions of the three ethnic groups on the theoretical variables in the sociocultural and personality systems was a major objective. A second major objective was to provide an account of individual differences by reference to the same theoretical framework. This involved a more direct test of the theory, an assessment of the direct relation of sociocultural and personality measures to the occurrence of deviant behavior.

Each of the measures in the sociocultural and personality systems was related, singly, to each of the multiple criterion measures of deviance and alcohol use. What these analyses showed was that, with some exceptions, the measures related in the direction which the theory implied but that the degree of relationship of each measure was generally small. Given our conceptualization of deviance as the complex outcome of both pressures and controls, low, single-measure correlations were not unexpected. The next step, therefore, was to deal simultaneously with multiple measures, and this was done by a pattern analysis procedure in which each individual was characterized by the “syndrome” of scores he had obtained with respect to measures of both pressures and controls. This pattern analysis procedure, which captures the intent of the theoretical interpretation, was more successful.

Considering the community as a whole, strong linear relations were shown to obtain between the sociocultural syndrome (which included measures of objective opportunity and social controls) and various criteria of deviance. The same was shown to be true for the relations between the personality pattern (which included measures of perceived opportunity, alienation, and personal controls) and deviance and drinking criteria. Most impressive, however, was the "field" pattern, which incorporated both sociocultural and personality measures (objective opportunity, social controls, perceived opportunity, and personal controls) into a single predictor pattern. The relation of the field pattern to the several criteria was shown to account for variance not accounted for by either the sociocultural or the personality patterns alone, and it tended consistently to yield the best prediction of the various deviance criteria in both the Community Survey Study and the High School Study. Treating the community adults as a whole and the high school students as a whole, the multivariable pattern analyses provided compelling evidence in support of the theoretical framework.

The final step in the direct assessment of the theory was to examine it, as above, *within* each of the ethnic groups. The pattern analyses retained the predictiveness they had shown for the community as a whole when they were applied within both the Anglo and Spanish groups, and for both sexes, but they were strongly attenuated in their ability to predict deviance within the Indian group. This attenuation seemed to be due in part to the high deviance rate characterizing the Indians and making differential within-group prediction extremely difficult. More will be said on this point in the discussion of limitations of the research.

To conclude this overview, a further point needs to be made. The measurement of deviance and deviance-prone behavior, such as heavy alcohol use, proved to be a task of great complexity, but one clearly meriting the attention it received. By retaining separate measures of various aspects of deviance and drinking behavior, we were able not only to assess the interrelations among them but also to use them as multiple, separate criteria in theory-testing. Further, by constructing a global index of deviance which combined various separate measures, we were able to approach most closely the kind of criterion the theory was directed at. This global deviance criterion was best and most consistently predicted by the sociocultural and personality measures.

In summary, these three studies in the Tri-Ethnic Research Project, the Community Survey Study of adults, the High School Study of adolescents, and the Socialization Study, yielded convergent, empirical support for the theoretical framework as an explanation of both group and individual differences in deviance and alcohol use. Such convergence suggests that inferences about the nature of deviance in this community, inferences of the sort contained in the theory, can be drawn with some degree of security.

Limitations of the Research

The preceding overview has focused upon the larger pattern of our findings. There were, however, a number of important limitations in our work stemming from the nature of the situation in which it was done, from our approach, and from our findings; these merit at least brief discussion at this point.

Perhaps the most salient question has to do with the character of the research context—a small, rural, southwestern community—and the constraints which it imposes upon generalizing from the findings. As with the study of any community, its representativeness of some universe is always in doubt, especially when the community has been selected, as in our case, for its particular ethnic composition. While there are obviously many other communities like the one in which we worked, it is difficult, on any sampling basis, to lay claim to inferences which go beyond its boundaries. This means, in the most severe terms, that our explanation of deviance applies only to this community, or perhaps to others which are demonstrably similar, and greater generalizability must wait upon extension and replication.

An aspect of this limitation which should be emphasized, and which illustrates the point, is that deviance in the research community cannot be said to be institutionalized in any formal sense. While there are informal peer groups, there do not appear to be gangs of the sort that characterize large urban centers, nor the formalized criminal organizations among adults frequently found in cities. Although the measures of deviance and deviance-prone behavior were comprehensive, they dealt with behavior which is most accurately described as only informally structured. The applicability of the findings is, therefore, in question where deviance can be shown to be a relatively institutionalized, formally supported and rewarded pattern of behavior.

A second major limitation has to do with the fact that the entire theory was not available at the outset of the research, but was in part developed during the process of investigation. This is most true of the social control formulations which, although considered from the beginning, were not specified in sufficient detail to guide the initial data collection. As the importance of social controls began to emerge, data already in hand were used to measure those concepts. While this was generally a feasible thing to do, it was obviously only poorly accomplished in certain respects—for example, in the measurement of opportunity to engage in deviance. Despite the support for the final social control formulations, support which obtained in the separate studies, their partially *post hoc* nature leaves this portion of the theory somewhat less securely established.

A third shortcoming is that certain of our measures simply did not work out. A primary example was the predictive failure of the internal-external control measure. A great deal of effort had gone into the development of this procedure, since the concept of internal-external control seemed theoretically important in linking personality with deviance, and since it was the kind of concept which could be readily coordinated with sociocultural variation. Its failure remains unclear to us, especially since it failed in both the High School and the Community Survey studies to show the expected relationships. These negative findings are not in accord with the success which the same or very similar measures have had in other studies (Rotter, 1966; Seeman, 1963; Wood, Wilson, Jessor, & Bogan, 1966), or with the importance which social-psychological analysis would assign to the concept. Further work is called for, and our data in this regard are disconcerting.

An additional shortcoming which we regret very much is our failure to explore in greater depth the role of peer groups and the impact of peer socialization. As informal influences conducing to or constraining against deviance, it is obvious they exert a strong influence. In the High School Study, sociometric data could have been employed to this end rather than serving simply as a criterion measure of deviance. In the Socialization Study, inquiry about peer associations could have been profitably undertaken. In both cases, the peer group network in which each youth is embedded would have been available for analysis, and the relation of peer support to the occurrence of deviance might have been better understood.

The inability of our approach to predict the particular *form* of deviant adaptation engaged in is a further limitation of note. The importance of measuring access to illegitimate means, especially the exposure to deviant role models component, was argued as the direction to take in coping with precisely this problem: with why, for example, one person may adapt to failure and frustration by mental illness, another by narcotics use, and a third by crime or heavy alcohol use. What would seem to be required is an analysis of exposure to various, alternative, deviant adaptations, an appraisal of the possibility of learning them through modeling, and an assessment of the conditions which may endow them differentially with the likelihood of success. In our own work, this type of detailed analysis was not made. Instead, we relied on a crude measure of exposure to any form of deviance, and this limitation precluded a contribution to the understanding of the selection of specific forms of deviance. Our approach, dealing with the *class* of deviant behaviors, was relevant to our concern with testing a general theory, but it meant that an important problem was not confronted.

The fact that our predictor measures in both the sociocultural and personality systems, when dealt with singly, generally had only low or moderate relationships to the criterion measures should also be commented on at this point. How much this reflects inadequate development of measures is difficult to say. Despite a tremendous expenditure of resources on the construction and refinement of measures, it is clear to us that we could have benefited from even more effort in this respect.

The recognition that, despite our efforts, the measures remained relatively crude, supported the decision to dichotomize the measures in devising the pattern analysis procedure. Although that decision seems to discard the possibility of greater discrimination, it does acknowledge the crudeness and attempts, by dichotomizing, to assure that variation on each predictor is securely established. It was the latter which was of primary concern to us in that our aim at this stage of theory development was to establish parameter *relevance* in prediction rather than to estimate parameter values.

A further shortcoming relates to the fact that the empirical findings do not clarify the issue of the conceptual unity of the separate theoretical structures posited within both the sociocultural and the personality systems. Alternative measures within each structure sometimes related better to measures in other structures than they did to each other; also, structures within one system sometimes related to structures in the other system which were *not* their conceptual analogue better than to the one that was. These data are not clear-cut: they support both a generality point of view and a specificity point of view about the functional unities implied by the separate structures. This issue will require further empirical and conceptual analysis. Empirically, there is a need to develop minimally overlapping measures which represent most precisely the conceptual content of each particular structure. Conceptually, the issue turns on the degree to which the structures within a system can be argued to be theoretically uncorrelated. The latter situation would be difficult to defend, either for the sociocultural system or the personality system, since the very notion of system implies a correlation among structures; and this is generally what we found. Whether relations within systems can obtain without jeopardizing the specificity of relations between analogous structures in different systems will only be known when further data are in hand. In the meantime, the theoretical structures postulated for the environment and for the person have thus far been of major heuristic value.

A final limitation to which attention must be called was the relatively poor prediction of deviance within the Indian group. While the pattern analyses showed effectiveness in accounting for variation in deviant behavior within both the Anglo and Spanish groups, only directional trends were obtained for the Indians. There are a number of possible explanations for this. It is possible, for example, that the interview procedures (and the reliance on non-Indian interviewers) were less appropriate to the Indian respondents than to the others in obtaining information on values, expectations, beliefs, and attitudes.

It is also possible that the measures were insufficiently sensitive to important factors differentially operative in the different ethnic groups. For example, while measures of values showed no ethnic group differences of any magnitude, it could be the case that measures focused upon other aspects of the orientation of minority groups to the dominant group could have revealed important differences. One such aspect, of obvious concern to the anthropologist, is acculturation. This concept did not enter directly into our theoretical framework; yet, a secondary analysis of some of our data interpreted in terms of the process of acculturation does seem to enhance prediction within both minority groups (see Graves, 1967). The analysis is *post hoc*, and the measures of acculturation are possibly tenuous, but the results attained are consistent and coherent, and they certainly suggest that the concept of acculturation may have utility in a community such as the one studied here.

One apparent problem in the attempt to account for differences in deviance within the Indian group is the fact of the high rate of Indian deviance, which makes discrimination an extremely difficult task. Given the general clustering of the Indian group at the upper end of the deviance criteria and at the deviance-prone end of the predictors, better prediction of individual differences within the Indian group would require predictors and criterion measures of much greater sensitivity. It is possible, too, that such a high rate of deviance, with the attendant patterning of learning and modeling which it implies, tends to make most of our predictors relatively unimportant determinants of deviant behavior. This difficulty in prediction within the Indian group should not, however, obscure the fact that, at the group level, an association between sociocultural and personality deviance proneness, on the one hand, and rates of deviant behavior, on the other, has been shown to exist.

The shortcomings of the research which have been noted do not constitute an exhaustive list. They are meant to represent some of the kinds of limitations which attenuate the strength of the findings and to alert the reader to the necessary caution in considering their implications, a few of which can be considered now.

Some Conclusions and Implications

Not too long ago, Henry Murray expressed the opinion that "no theoretical system constructed on the psychological level will be adequate until it has been embraced by and intermeshed with a cultural-sociological system" (1959, p. 20). At the most general level, this view was a starting point for us, and the outcome of our work impels us to return to it as a conclusion. The explanatory usefulness of a field theory of behavior has been shown to extend beyond the limits of its psychological and sociocultural component systems. When the latter are "intermeshed," certain previously recalcitrant problems become more docile, problems such as why everyone at the same social location does not behave the same way, or why the epidemiology of certain behaviors is patterned in a particular way in the social structure. Beyond these practical consequences, however, there is the fundamental gain of being able, through reliance upon a field theoretical system, to generate more detailed intelligibility about social behavior.

To make this point about the over-all theory is not to diminish the importance of the particular concepts within the embracing systems. Conclusions about certain of the concepts we have used can, as a matter of fact, be drawn with a fair degree of confidence. It is clear, for example, that the notion of *expectation* constitutes one of our most powerful concepts for describing persons with respect to deviance proneness. Differences in values were relatively minor, whether those values were defined in the common language referring to success or whether they were defined in motivationally relevant terms. What emerged as crucially important were differences in expectation for achieving what was valued. That expectations play a central role in the selective course of human behavior seems clear from the data. This conclusion has greater impact when it is realized that the measures of expectation were conceptually remote from the behavior at issue; unlike another of the psychological measures, tolerance of deviance, which also turned out to be an important predictor, but which dealt directly with deviance, the expectations measures never implicated deviance in the actual measurement procedure.

The conclusion about the important role of expectations in social behavior is in accord with the literature and would seem to have pervasive implications for efforts to deal with problem behavior. Social intervention focused upon raising expectations that socially desirable behavior can lead successfully to valued goals would be a tactic consonant with those implications. That such expectations follow, in part at least, from the position occupied in the opportunity structure is suggested by the research and makes the latter a prime target for concentration in organizing efforts at remediation.

To move to a consideration of the concepts employed to describe the sociocultural environment, certainly *social controls* have emerged as central. The critical part played by social controls was nowhere clearer than in the differentiation it yielded between the two minority ethnic groups. Both groups are subjected to strong pressures toward deviance, yet the Spanish, embedded in a persisting structure of religious, family, and interpersonal sanctions, contribute far less to the deviance rates than the Indians, for whom the control structure is fragmented or weak. The meaning of controls in our research is in large part the degree to which a person is mapped into solidary groups that reward conforming behavior, punish departures from group norms, and provide relatively few models for deviance. Other things equal, the strengthening of family and both formal and informal group ties would seem to be relevant to efforts toward reducing deviance.

The latter point is probably also relevant to increasing the degree of normative consensus or agreement about what is appropriate in the way of behavior. The research has demonstrated the possibility of relatively direct measurement of anomie and, although the data derive, unfortunately, from only one study, suggests that such lack of normative consensus may be relevant to deviance. The strengthening of social ties, and the corollary development of interpersonal communication, may be as important in reducing anomie as in strengthening social controls.

The analyses of deviance have been instructive in themselves. The use of multiple raters (for example, teachers, or peers) and multiple sources of data (for example, self-reports, records, teacher ratings, or peer nominations) enable increased reliability and convergent validity to overcome the possible shortcomings of self-reports. It should be noted, in regard to the latter, that our own experience justifies reliance upon self-report data, especially where the concern is with rank-ordering a group of subjects on degree of deviance. The convergence, in our research, between self-report data and external criteria of deviance was impressive.

The findings about alcohol use make the complexity of deviance most evident. Comprehensive understanding of alcohol use required knowledge of how it was learned, the context of its use, the amount drunk, the meaning or psychological functions of drinking, and the consequences of its use. Two persons drinking moderate amounts of alcohol may be doing so in very different ways: one by himself, as a way of overcoming a feeling of being nervous or tense; and the other in a group, as a way of expressing his feeling of community with his companions. The difference between these two patterns is not only likely to have different consequences but to be differentially related to sociocultural and personality pressures and controls as well.

What the research has indicated is that at least several aspects of alcohol use are explicable in terms of the sociocultural and personality concepts in the over-all scheme. This was most apparent where the alcohol use was heavy and for personal-effects, problem-solving reasons (although the scheme did show predictiveness, even for the amount of alcohol drunk). The demonstration that excessive alcohol use is related to differential pressures and controls, both sociocultural and personality, has important implications, not only for understanding this form of problem behavior but also for possible remedial measures.

A final implication of the research requiring mention has to do with the meaning of the concept of ethnicity. Our work has contributed to a social-psychology of ethnicity or ethnic status. Instead of dealing with ethnic status in terms of some set of unique traits or in terms of a peculiar cultural legacy distinctive of a particular group, we have dealt with it as representing a position in social-psychological space. A unitary set of sociocultural, personality, and behavior measures has been applied to all three ethnic groups. The result of this approach was an analysis of ethnic status in the language of the theoretical scheme. Thus, what it means to be an Indian in this community is to have limited opportunity, to be confronted by relatively pervasive anomie, to be subject to weak social controls, and the like. Ethnic status, then, is merely a descriptive term, but one probabilistically implying a bundle of theoretical attributes.

This interpretation of the concept of ethnicity is analogous to what Oscar Lewis has urged with respect to another descriptive concept: poverty. In developing the notion of "the culture of poverty," Lewis has gathered together a number of traits often considered to represent distinctive characteristics of ethnic, national, or regional groups and has argued that these characteristics are:

> "...both an adaptation and a reaction of the poor to their marginal position in a class-stratified, highly individuated, capitalistic society. It represents an effort to cope with feelings of hopelessness and despair that arise from the realization by the members of the marginal communities in these societies of the improbability of their achieving success in terms of the prevailing values and goals." (1966, p. 21).

Lewis' distinction between poverty and the culture of poverty is analogous to the distinction we are suggesting between ethnic status and the social-psychology of ethnic status. It happens that poverty and ethnic or marginal status often go together; that is probably what accounts for the fact that the content of Lewis' culture of poverty and the content of our social-psychology of ethnic status have so much in common.

The implications of this discussion seem important. They suggest that the deviance rates of the three ethnic groups characterize them not by virtue of their ethnic status, but largely by virtue of their social-psychological status; place Anglos in the situation of Indians, and deviance rates should increase markedly. Such a view departs sharply from that part of the community psychology which, for example, considers deviance and drunkenness an inherently Indian trait. Further, this view would seem important in any considerations of change; insofar as the problem is seen not as a problem of ethnicity but as a problem of the attributes associated with it, the latter become the obvious target of change efforts.

Finally, this perspective provides a rationale for considering, as a single unit or as a whole, communities which are made up of different ethnic groups. Precisely this has been done in some of the major analyses presented here. Although the groups are descriptively different, the rationale suggests that they can be treated homogeneously in terms of their position on a set of variables applicable to all members of the community, variables which, in essence, summarize much of the social and psychological meaning of ethnic status.

A final word: Our work has captured, obviously, neither the quality of daily life nor the succession of events which pattern the course of time in the community; that task belongs to the sensitive ethnographer. Instead, the path we chose to follow was an abstract one, and it is now possible to see where it has led. The ideas developed and the data generated have given us a beginning sense of understanding. Hopefully, they may have application to other social problems as well and, ultimately, may contribute in a small way to the amelioration of the human condition. It would be difficult, at this stage, to ask more of behavioral science.

References

Cloward, R. A., & Ohlin, L. E. (1961). *Delinquency and opportunity*. New York: Free Press.

Graves, T. D. (1967). Acculturation, access, and alcohol in a tri-ethnic community. *American Anthropologist, 69*(3–4), 306–321.

Jessor, R., Graves, T. D., Hanson, R. C., & Jessor, S. L. (1968). Chapter 13: Overview and appraisal of theory and findings. In R. Jessor, T. D. Graves, R. C. Hanson, & S. L. Jessor (Eds.), *Society, personality, and deviant behavior: A study of a tri-ethnic community* (pp. 407–421). New York: Holt, Rinehart and Winston.

Lewis, O. (1966). The culture of poverty. *Scientific American, 215*(4), 19–25.

Merton, R. K. (1957). *Social theory and social structure* (Rev. and enl. ed.). New York: Free Press.

Murray, H. A. (1959). Preparations for the scaffold of a comprehensive system. In S. Koch (Ed.), *Psychology: A study of a science* (Vol. 3, pp. 7–54). New York: McGraw-Hill.

Rotter, J. B. (1954). *Social learning and clinical psychology*. Englewood Cliffs, NJ: Prentice-Hall.

Rotter, J. B. (1966). Generalized expectancies for internal versus external control of reinforcement. *Psychological Monographs* (Vol. 80, Whole No. 609). Washington, DC: American Psychological Association.

Seeman, M. (1963). Alienation and social learning in a reformatory. *American Journal of Sociology, 69*(3), 270–284.

Wood, B. S., Wilson, G. G., Jessor, R., & Bogan, J. B. (1966). Troublemaking behavior in a correctional institution: Relationship to inmates' definition of their situation. *American Journal of Orthopsychiatry, 36*(5), 795–802.

Chapter 4
Problem Behavior Theory and Adolescent Development

Richard Jessor and Shirley L. Jessor

In this chapter (Jessor, R. & Jessor, S.L., 1977, Chap. 12) we conclude a rather long odyssey, a quest for understanding of problem behavior and development in a segment of American youth. The chapter provides an opportunity to take stock—to note the limitations as well as the advantages of the approach we followed, to review what has been learned, and to consider some issues that have important implications for a final perspective on the research as a whole.

The basic aim of the study was to evaluate the adequacy of Problem Behavior Theory and to examine the extent to which such a social-psychological framework could yield a sensible account of the variation in problem behavior—both cross-sectional and longitudinal—that is evident among youth. The approach, in brief, was to derive measures from the theory, to enlist the participation of young people in high school and college, and to follow the lives of those participants over a significant number of years. In addition to allowing for an appraisal of the usefulness of the theory, the approach made it possible to witness, at the same time, the shape and direction of psychosocial growth and development.

That Problem Behavior Theory has received a good measure of empirical support in this application is apparent. For both males and females, in both high school and college, with regard to both cross-sectional and longitudinal data, and for both problem and conventional behavior, the findings tend to be consistent and coherent,

Reprinted with permission from:
Jessor, R., & Jessor, S. L. (1977). Chapter 12: "A final perspective." In R. Jessor & S. L. Jessor, *Problem behavior and psychosocial development: A longitudinal study of youth* (pp. 231–248). New York: Academic Press.

R. Jessor (✉)
Institute of Behavioral Science, University of Colorado at Boulder, Boulder, CO 80309, USA
e-mail: jessor@Colorado.edu

S.L. Jessor
(deceased)

R. Jessor, *The Origins and Development of Problem Behavior Theory*,
Advancing Responsible Adolescent Development,
DOI 10.1007/978-3-319-40886-6_4

often substantial in magnitude, and instructive in their patterning. Some review of this outcome, as well as the areas in which support was meager or lacking, will be useful, but a more reasonable judgment of its significance can be made if the liabilities and assets of the study are catalogued first.

An Appraisal of the Approach

Although most of the limitations of this investigation have been noted earlier, several are important enough to warrant further mention. First, the samples of high school and college youth who participated in the research cannot be considered representative of the populations from which they were drawn. The initial loss from the designated random sampling was large, and the nature of the bias that may have been generated by that loss was impossible to measure. In all likelihood, the result was a somewhat more conventional sample of participants. Subsequent attrition over the 4 years of testing was modest in both studies; while examination of the dropouts did not reveal them to differ in a major way from those who remained, their loss could have been an additional source of bias. Finally, the community itself was a highly selected one—a small university city with a largely middle-class, white population. Clearly, the generality of inference from this study is constrained by these sampling limitations. Fortunately, there was wide variation on nearly all the measures among those who participated and the number of participants was large enough to permit a variety of partitionings—both facts essential to our primary concern with theory testing *within* the samples. Further, the generality of the findings receives support from other studies of other samples, including a study of a national sample (these will be commented on later).

A second limitation derives from the design itself, namely, the absence of a control group for the assessment of testing effects or the degree to which longitudinal change on the various measures can be considered an outcome of the procedure of making repeated measurements. Such a control is important in longitudinal research and should be implemented wherever feasible. Its absence in our study required that a set of arguments be adduced to protect the changes reported from vulnerability to a testing-effects interpretation. One of the main ones points to the consistency between the direction of change over time and the direction of the *initial* differences among the three age cohorts in the High School Study. Unfortunately, the absence of a cohort-sequential design in the College Study precluded that argument from being made for those data.

The nearly exclusive reliance upon self-report measures—with the exception of the Family Interview Study and the acquisition of academic records—could be considered a third major limitation of the research. The validity of self-report is always open to challenge, and the topic has even engaged controversy of an epistemological nature. Our own position is straightforward: For certain kinds of information there is simply no alternative to reliance on self-report. Procedures exist for maximizing veridicality. In the earlier Tri-Ethnic Study, a very large and costly effort was made to obtain independent measures (e.g., court records, teacher ratings, and peer nominations) to validate self-reports; we found, in the end, that they did not alter the basic self-report findings. A similar conclusion was arrived at by Elliott and Voss (1974) in their longitudinal study of delinquency and dropout among high school youth. That independent measures are a salutary complement to a questionnaire study is beyond argument—not so much, in our view, as a validity check on self-reports but as a source of additional, and perhaps different, kinds of information. Had it been feasible, we would have included intensive interviewing of the participants, and their friends as well, solicited autobiographies, and obtained regular information from their parents. Given the necessity to limit data collection to questionnaires in this study, our effort was directed to ensuring the quality and enhancing the validity of self-reporting.

From the perspective of testing the developmental implications of Problem Behavior Theory, the omission of a key measure constitutes a fourth limitation: our failure to map and to measure directly the age-graded norms that had been assumed in the formulation of the concept of transition proneness. Theoretically, the age grading of norms about transition behaviors is an important facet of the social environment of youth, and measurement of such norms should be high on any agenda for developmental research. In a follow-up study of a national sample of youth that is currently under way, we have included measures of the age grading of norms, and the data from those items will be of considerable interest. Nevertheless, their omission from the present investigation has prevented a key theoretical linkage from being empirically established.

In the area of data analysis, two limitations deserve acknowledgement. The first is our failure to carry the analysis of longitudinal change on the theoretical measures beyond the univariate level. The ultimate need is for a multivariate approach to individual *patterns* of change, for example, through profile analysis or the establishment of change types (see Block, 1971). Although an initial effort was made to explore a system for typing multivariate change patterns, the work was not carried forward and remains a task for the future. The other limitation stems from our reliance upon multiple regression analysis for assessing the multivariate account yielded by the variables in Problem Behavior Theory. Because the model that underlies multiple regression is linear and additive, it does not reflect the interactive or nonadditive relations that may exist. In that regard, it may not constitute the best procedure for testing the field theoretical perspective that informs Problem Behavior Theory.

Mention of other limitations—for example, lack of study of the school context, the 12-month interval between testings that made it difficult to deal more precisely with the time of onset of problem behaviors, and the fact that several of our variables simply didn't "work"—would not exhaust the list. Our aim in describing them has been to indicate our awareness that in some degree they constrain the inferences that can be drawn from the research.

It is important to emphasize, however, that none of the limitations is considered serious enough to undermine the study or to jeopardize its major aims. Such a statement can be made because the shortcomings of the approach were balanced by its advantages. Foremost among the assets of the approach is its reliance upon and involvement with theory. As a theory-oriented study, this research differs from much social-psychological research on youth. Theory helps to minimize inferential ambiguity by permitting the logical derivation of measures and by organizing the observations in a logically consistent fashion. Beyond that, theory provides a framework for explanation. In addition to these logical advantages, the substantive nature of Problem Behavior Theory had an important influence on the research approach. It fostered a comprehensiveness and a differentiation of measurement. The large number of attributes assessed and their organization into structures and systems yielded a multivariate measurement map with considerably greater explanatory impact than would otherwise have been achieved.

At the design level, several assets of the approach merit comment. The parallel studies at the high school level and the college level provided an opportunity for theory testing at two quite different developmental levels and permitted the observation of important differences as well as similarities. The multiple cohorts in the High School Study extended the generality of the findings by revealing consistencies, especially in longitudinal change, among these independent samples of younger adolescents. And the inclusion of males and females enabled a further examination of generality, this time across the sexes at both developmental levels. Finally, the employment of as many as four annual testing occasions ensured that a period of time long enough to be of developmental significance at this stage of the life trajectory had been covered. Together, these facets of the research design contributed unusual possibilities for the replication or cross-validation of specific findings—across age, school level, sex, and four waves of time—and it is such replication that ultimately provides conviction about scientific inference.

The approach to measurement would seem to be another advantage of the study worth noting. Reliance throughout was on theory-derived, structured measures that had been psychometrically developed and, for the most part, construct validated in prior research. Such an approach maximizes the reliability of findings as well as their interpretability, and it is especially crucial in studies where time extension and repeated measurement are involved.

Another advantage of the research approach was the inclusion of multiple criterion measures of problem and conventional behaviors. The bulk of contemporary research in this area tends to be behavior specific, focusing on drinking, or drug use, or sex, or delinquency. This pattern reflects not only the vagaries of societal concern but the topical interests and career commitments of researchers, and even the mission orientation of the separate funding agencies. Nevertheless, a behavior-specific focus can be misleading. It fails to reveal that other behaviors may function as alternatives and that the empirical findings may be general rather than specific. Our measurement of a behavior *system* permitted direct examination of generality, allowed for the replication of Problem Behavior Theory across phenotypically diverse behaviors, and enabled a demonstration of discriminant validity in relation to such conventional behavior as church attendance.

The assets are reminders of points that have already been made. Their importance derives from the implications they have for the scope and depth of the empirical assessment of Problem Behavior Theory. All of these implications converge on the concern with "minimizing inferential ambiguity," a methodological objective elaborated in the earlier Tri-Ethnic Study (see Jessor et al., 1968, Chap. 6). In light of the advantages discussed, and despite the limitations noted, the research approach employed in this study would seem able to sustain a good deal of confidence in the findings that emerged.

A Review of the Major Findings

Since the research results have been presented in detail earlier, our aim in this section is to highlight the more general aspects of the empirical outcome. First, with respect to Problem Behavior Theory, its usefulness has been significantly reinforced. The magnitude of the account it provided for variation in problem behavior was in many cases substantial—about 50% of the variance in the multiple problem behavior index, for example—and the generality of the account was evident in relation to a number of specific behaviors, including involvement with marijuana and general deviance (among others). Discriminant validity for the theory was established by the demonstration that its variables related to conventional behavior in a direction opposite to their relation to problem behavior. And finally, the effectiveness of the theory in accounting for development and change in behavior served to buttress its cross-sectional utility. Taken together as an organized set of concepts, Problem Behavior Theory has emerged as a relevant framework for social-psychological research. In addition to its overall contribution, however, its component systems and structures have furthered an understanding of the factors in the person and in the environment that mediate variation in action.

In relation to those component systems and their structures, the results were of interest. To begin with the behavior system, several key findings warrant emphasis. First, the prevalence of what we have called problem behaviors was substantial at the college level and, while much lower, sizable at the high school level. In the High School Study, for example, more than a third of the youth had had some experience with marijuana, and a third had experienced sexual intercourse by the Year IV testing. Second, the findings provided strong support for the general concept of problem behavior by revealing an interrelatedness—a syndrome character—among the diverse behaviors subsumed by the concept, and their covariation was placed in sharper relief by their inverse relation to conventional behavior. Not all the behaviors co-varied, activism being one exception, and the syndrome character was much stronger at the high school than at the college level, but relatedness among problem behaviors was quite clear in general. A third point about the behavior system is that problem and conventional behavior are not mutually exclusive and may co-occur in the same individual; this finding reinforces our concern to reserve those adjectives, "problem" and "conventional," for behavior and not for persons.

With regard to the personality system, the most important empirical outcome was the demonstration of its significant role in the occurrence of problem behavior in youth. Regression analyses of personality system measures in the High School System yielded multiple correlations beyond .50 for the multiple problem behavior index and for measures of marijuana use and general deviance, for example. (The theoretical role of personality is one of the issues to return to shortly.) The finding about the personality system that seems to be next in importance is the differential effectiveness of its component structures. As a general statement, personal controls appear to be most influential in relation to the set of problem behaviors, motivational-instigations are next, and personal beliefs are least (and for the most part weak). This importance of personality factors of a cognitive, moral ideological nature is noteworthy. Third, the variable that most consistently and generally represented the contribution of each structure to the explanatory account was the independence-achievement value discrepancy in the motivational-instigation structure, social criticism in the personal belief structure, and attitudinal tolerance of deviance in the personal control structure (disregarding, for the moment, the highly proximal disjunction measures in the latter). As a cluster, the triad suggests that proneness to problem behavior rests upon a personality pattern that implicates unconventionality.

In relation to the personality system as a whole, the adolescent who is less likely to engage in problem behavior is one who values academic achievement and expects to do well academically, who is not concerned much with independence, who treats society as unproblematic rather than as deserving of criticism and reshaping, who maintains a religious involvement and is more uncompromising about transgression, and who finds little that is positive in problem behavior relative to the negative consequences of engaging in it. The adolescent who is more likely to engage in problem behavior shows an opposite personality pattern—a concern with personal autonomy, a relative lack of interest in the goals of conventional institutions (such as school and church), a jaundiced view of the larger society, and a more tolerant attitude about transgression.

The most salient finding about the perceived environment system is the powerful contribution it made to the explanation of variation in problem behavior. In the High School Study, it yielded multiple correlations close to .70 with the problem behavior index, for both males and females. In most cases the contribution of the perceived environment system was greater than that of the personality system. Insight into the likely reason for this prepotency derives from the findings about the two structures of the perceived environment; it is apparent that the proximal structure carries most of the explanatory weight, and it is the inclusion of proximal variables in the perceived environment system that enables it to outweigh the more distal variables of the personality system. More will be said about this issue shortly.

Within the distal structure of the perceived environment, the variables that indicate whether a youth is parent oriented or peer oriented are the most significant. In the proximal structure, the variables referring to peer models and support for problem behavior are most important. Together they suggest the character of a problem-prone environment; adolescents who are likely to engage in problem behavior perceive less compatibility between the expectations that their parents and their friends hold for them, they acknowledge greater influence of friends relative to parents, they perceive greater support for problem behavior among their friends, and they have more friends who provide models for engaging in problem behavior.

With respect to the field-theoretical (or interactionist) stance that has been built into the social-psychological framework of Problem Behavior Theory, the findings have strengthened our conviction that a more exhaustive account of behavior requires joint reliance on person and environment variables. Two aspects of the results bear on this conclusion. First, in most of the field pattern runs of the uniform multivariate analysis procedure there was an increment in the multiple correlation over the correlation for the separate personality or perceived environment run. Although the increment was usually small, this is not surprising since the two component systems have a good deal of shared variance. That they nevertheless contribute unique variance to the field pattern run is the second aspect of the results that needs mention. The final step-wise multiple regression equation for the six different problem behaviors and for the two conventional behaviors always included at least one personality measure and one perceived environment measure. This was true for males and females in Year IV of the High School Study. It constitutes important support for the field theory perspective since it reveals the joint role of the personality and perceived environment systems in the explanation of problem behavior.

Since the developmental results are relevant to an issue to be discussed shortly—the causal structure of the findings—only the descriptive trends will be noted here, and again the summary focuses on the High School Study. The trajectories that were plotted from the four annual measurements suggest a variety of growth trends in each system of Problem Behavior Theory and for both sexes. These developmental changes include growth of independence, decline in traditional ideology related to achievement value and to society as a whole, assumption of a more relativistic and more tolerant morality, attenuation of the hold of conventional norms and controls such as those embodied in religion and the family, increase in orientation toward peers and in reliance on them as a reference group, ecological increase in the prevalence of models and supports for transgression, and increase in problem behavior itself. These findings are of major interest for several reasons. They are based on longitudinal data rather than inferred from cross-sectional samples varying in age; they describe aspects of the course of normal development, the aggregate direction of change in our normal samples of high school youth; and, of theoretical relevance, they suggest that the normal course of developmental change in adolescence is in the direction of greater problem proneness. This latter point implies that problem behavior may be viewed, at least in part, as an aspect of growing up. This is a notion we will return to later.

In this review of the major findings the generalizations have been large and the exceptions have been ignored. That imbalance can be righted by reminding ourselves of the more important qualifications that need to be made in regard to the reach of the theory and the effectiveness of the measures. Our reliance on the High School Study in the foregoing summary was not an accident; rather, it was because the results were strongest at that level, and while the College Study data tend to be supportive, they were considerably weaker. More specifically, the motivational-instigation variables of the personality system have little relevance to problem behavior at the college level, and the distal structure of the perceived environment is also unimportant. Personal controls remain effective, however, and the proximal environment continues to be influential. This difference is illuminating in that the social psychology of problem behavior takes a somewhat different shape at the later developmental level than at the earlier one, a fact that would have remained hidden without the two studies. It may be that the higher prevalence levels of problem behavior at the college level and the more accepting age norms about engaging in such behavior at that level make it less of a normative departure. Under such circumstances, instigation would seem to be less necessary, and the main source of variation would likely derive from controls.

Between the two sexes, Problem Behavior Theory was somewhat more effective for the females. The reasons for this may be similar to those applied to the difference between the two developmental levels. One of the legacies of sex-role differentiation is to view problem behavior in females as more of a normative departure than in males. To the extent to which this is true, it may make for greater relevance of the theory to females. Overall, however, the results for both sexes, especially at the high school level, were convergent.

Although the theory showed generality across behaviors, note should be taken of its limited success in regard to activism in the problem behavior structure and academic achievement or grade-point average in the conventional behavior structure. Activism was not well predicted and tended not to co-vary with the other problem behaviors. While there were measurement problems with activism and while it fluctuated over time in a nonsystematic fashion, we are uncertain of the reasons for its refractory role. Grade-point average was also poorly predicted (except by the very proximal measure of expectations for academic achievement), nor did it co-vary with the other conventional behavior, church attendance. Given the indirectness of its interpretation as a conventional behavior, given the role played by ability in academic achievement, and given grading practices that shift with grade in school, this outcome was not surprising.

One other behavior area should be mentioned, namely, problem drinking. The results presented earlier showed that there was only limited support for the personality system measures in relation to problem drinker status, an exception being the personal control variable of tolerance of deviance. This should not be taken as a general failure of the theory to account for problem drinking, however. The overall multivariate analysis yields multiple correlations close to .60 in the High School Study, and a test of the personality system in an earlier year yielded better results, even in that domain, than those reported for Year IV. Part of the difficulty with the measure of problem drinker status may have been that the criterion definition was too modest.

Finally, in this set of qualifications about the findings, note should be taken of several variables in the conceptual framework that were consistently weak or showed only meager relations to problem behavior. Value on affection and expectation for affection are two motivational-instigation variables in this group. The item content of these measures stressed what might be called peer popularity rather than intimacy and affectional closeness, and social popularity was not a widely endorsed value at the turn of the decade. Perhaps this is part of the reason for its poor showing. Three other variables also should be included: self-esteem, alienation, and internal-external locus of control—all belonging to the personal belief structure.

Psychometric difficulties with the latter two were apparent in their lack of unidimensionality, but the main problem with all three was their failure to show consistent linkages with variation in behavior. A theoretical issue is raised by this failure and its resolution is another task for the future.

One other fact should be recorded. Our findings are consonant with those reported by a variety of other investigators, some working independently and others relying on concepts or measures from our work. Kandel's (1978) review of research on youthful drug use emphasizes such convergence; the findings of Elliott and Voss (1974) on delinquency, of Sadava on drug use (1973), of Braucht (1974) on a variety of problem behaviors, and of Nesselroade and Baltes (1974) on developmental change are other examples of areas of commonality of results.

Most important, however, is a recent national sample survey of 13,000 high school youth (Rachal, Williams, Brehm, Cavanaugh, Moore, & Eckerman, 1975) that employed a number of the measures from our study; the findings turn out to be very consistent with those in our research. For example, an overall multiple correlation between a similar set of predictors and marijuana involvement was .74 and .75 for males and females, respectively (see Chase & Jessor, 1977). In our Year IV data in the High School Study, the comparable correlations were .76 and .77. For problem drinker status, the national sample multiple correlations were .59 and .60 for males and females respectively (see Donovan & Jessor, 1976); in our High School Study, the comparable Year IV correlations were .59 and .45. Further support is apparent in recent analyses of general deviant behavior in the national sample (see Donovan, 1977). These findings are especially important to us because, unlike ours, they are based on a large national sample that contains wide variation on socioeconomic, ethnic, regional, and rural-urban characteristics. It suggests that our findings may not be confined to the highly selected community in which they were gathered and, at least at the level of theoretical relations, that they may have considerable generality.

A Consideration of Some General Issues

A number of issues remain to be considered in light of what has been learned from this study. In this section we raise them briefly and try to draw out some of their implications for research and theory and for youth and society.

The Causal Structure of the Findings

The most elusive and recalcitrant of all objectives in behavioral science, especially in field research, is the establishment of causal relationships. Causal inference is ultimately a matter of logic and theory rather than an automatic product of a particular research design, even one that is longitudinal. While causality lies beyond demonstration, conviction about it can be strengthened by the organization of multiple converging research strategies. Listing the 10 strategies employed in the present research can serve as a way of summarizing where we have arrived in relation to the causal relevance of Problem Behavior Theory.

The first research strategy was the reliance on theory; the second was the employment of theory-derived and construct-validated measures; the third was the provision in the design for numerous replications and cross-validations of findings. The fourth was the demonstration of theoretical relationships among the variables at a cross-section in time, and the fifth was the exploration of socialization antecedents of the attributes in the framework. These five strategies did not require longitudinal design, whereas the five that follow did.

The sixth strategy was the description of change over time, in both the "predictor" and "criterion" measures, and the establishment of theoretical consonance in the two sets of changes. The seventh was forecasting the onset of behavior over an interval of time; the eighth was the demonstration of interindividual differences in development that were systematically linked to the time of onset of various behaviors; the ninth (reported in earlier papers) was the demonstration, by residualized gain scores, of a greater amount of change on the theoretical variables when a change in behavior occurred than when it did not; and the tenth strategy was the use of cross-lagged panel correlations to indicate directionality of influence in the predictor-criterion associations.

Some of these strategies are discussed elsewhere (Jessor & Jessor, 1978) and, with the exception of the last one, have been commented upon earlier. The contribution of the cross-lagged panel correlation strategy can be illustrated briefly in Fig. 4.1 (taken from some ongoing work with our data by John Finney). Since Kenny (1975) suggests that a cross-lagged difference ideally should replicate across different time lags and different groups of participants, we have presented 3-wave data in Fig. 4.1, and for males and females separately. The directionality suggested by the high school data in Fig. 4.1 is clearly from personality (attitudinal tolerance of deviance) to behavior (marijuana behavior involvement). This inference is drawn from the pattern of lagged correlations, those that belong to the diagonal lines in the figure. In all three cases for each sex, the magnitude of the correlation is greater in the personality-behavior direction than in the behavior-personality direction during the same interval. Interpretation of cross-lagged analyses is, of course, more complex than this (see Kenny's discussion, cited above), but our concern here is simply to present the kind of contribution this strategy can make.

Taken together, the 10 strategies have generated a high degree of convergence, and the logical structure they comprise is coherent. Consonance of results from the separate strategies—for example, the commonality between the variables that are associated cross-sectionally with problem behavior and those that predict its onset over time—makes for strong conviction about the *explanatory relevance* of the variables. But it needs to be emphasized that none of the strategies, separately or together, does more than document an association, even where temporal order is known, and therefore *causal influence* has not been demonstrated. What the multiple, converging strategies have yielded is a strong sense that the theoretical variables are closely involved in the processes that surround the occurrence of problem

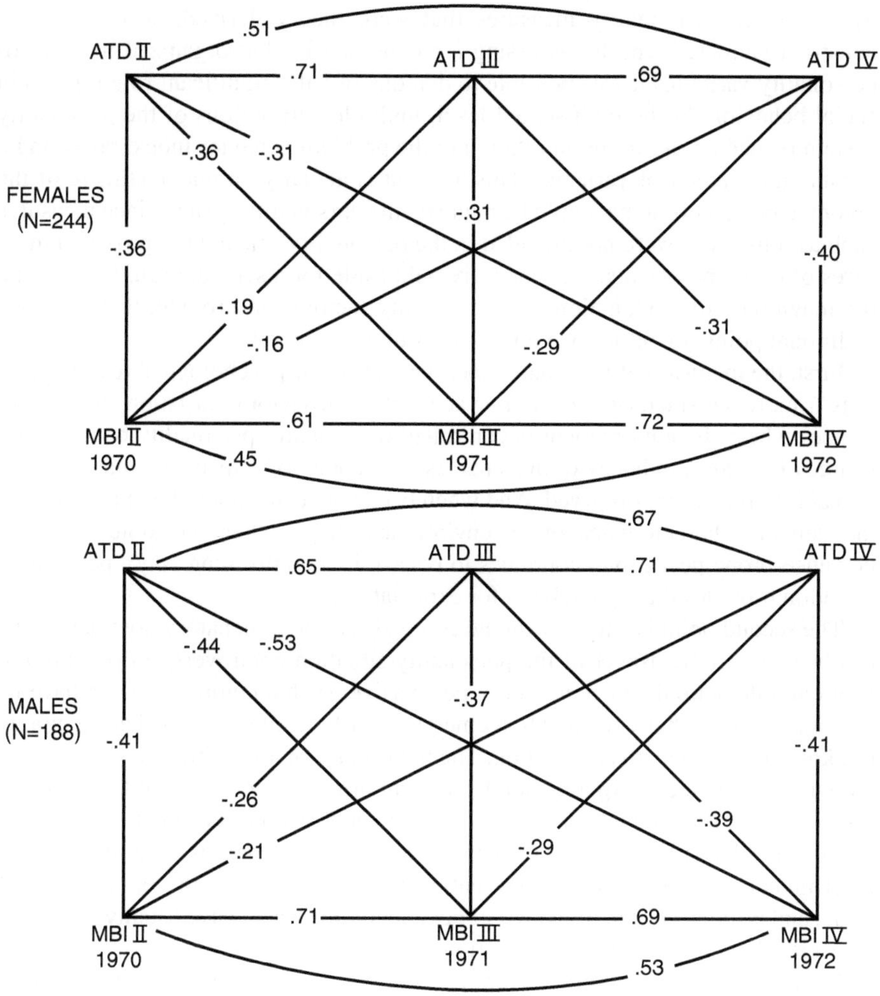

Fig. 4.1 Cross-lagged panel correlations for attitudinal tolerance of deviance (ATD) and marijuana behavior involvement (MBI) for Years II, III, and IV, High School Study

behavior in youth and are relevant to its development over time. Were it not for these convergent strategies, that conviction and that sense of relevance would have remained tenuous and delicate.

The Role of Personality. In recent years, in psychology at least, interest in personality has languished; its conceptual status had been widely challenged and its empirical utility had been severely depreciated. One of our aims in this research was to contribute to a revitalization of interest in personality as an explanatory system. By conceptualizing personality at a cognitive-social level, by formulating personality variables that have logical linkages to the environment and to behavior, by employing personality measures that were theory derived, structured, and construct validated, and by assessing a comprehensive but organized network of personality variables it was possible to demonstrate the significant role it plays in social behavior. At the high school level, multiple correlations of the personality system reached close to .60 in relation to the problem behavior index, providing a substantial account of variance. This account is actually an underestimate of the potential contribution that could be made by the personality system since measures such as religiosity were not included in the personality run and the proximal measures of drug and sex disjunctions were held aside for a separate run. But beyond the magnitude of explanation that personality factors can provide, there are two additional points to emphasize on the basis of our research.

First, the inclusion of personality measures in social-psychological research permits a more satisfactory *explanatory* account of behavioral variation. In circumstances where the environment is controlled or standard, personality constitutes a source of variance in behavior that enables an account to be made of whatever individual differences are observed. And when behavior seems not to be in accord with the demand characteristics of an environment (e.g., when an adolescent in a deviance-prone peer group continues to behave in a conforming way), personality variation provides the logical basis for explanation.

The second point has to do with the competition for explanatory dominance that has been a chronic aspect of the personality-situation controversy in psychology. From an interactionist or field theory perspective, such a competition can have no meaning. But another consideration emerges clearly from our work that has not, to our knowledge, been given attention. The importance of a variable or a system—the amount of variance it explains in a behavioral criterion—depends in large part on how proximal it is to the behavior, rather than whether it is a personality or a situational variable. In the disputes over whether the environment is a more important determinant than personality, no attention has been given to the proximal-distal issue, and critiques of the weakness of personality measures have usually addressed measures that are very distal from action.

We can illustrate the point we are making with our data on the multiple problem behavior index. In the High School Study the multivariate personality run yielded multiple correlations of .57 and .58 for males and females, respectively. If we want to ask whether the correlations for the perceived environment are better or worse than this, the answer is that *it depends on which part of the perceived environment is considered.* The multiple correlations for the *proximal* structure are better, .69 and .69 for the two sexes, but the multiple correlations for the *distal* structure are worse, .36 and .39. Exactly the same pattern holds at the college level. The personality run correlations are .29 and .41 for males and females; the correlations for the proximal structure of the perceived environment are again better, .61 and .64, while those for the distal structure are again worse, .25 and .23. No discussion of the relative explanatory contribution of personality and environmental factors can be meaningful without recognition of the necessity to consider the proximal-distal dimension.

We touched on this issue in relation to the proximal character of the measures in the personal control structure, and in Jessor and Jessor (1973) in regard to the differentiation of the perceived environment. The findings in the present study have been especially illuminating because we have maintained an analytic separation between the personality system and the perceived environment system, and because of the differentiated structures within each system. On both logical and empirical grounds, the importance of personality as an explanatory system in social-psychological research has been strengthened by the outcome of this study.

The Role of the Environment

Since the environment issue received consideration in the preceding section, only one point will be raised here. It has to do with our choice to focus upon the perceived environment rather than, say, the sociocultural environment or the demographic environment, which are more independent of the actor. In analyses of the demographic data that were collected, relations with problem behavior variation were generally meager and inconsequential. Unfortunately, the limited range of socioeconomic and ethnic differences in the research community made for an unsatisfactory test. Where better tests were possible, however, the outcome was not very different. For example, Elliott and Voss (1974) indicate that in their data delinquent behavior does not appear to be related to social class or ethnic origins; and in her review of research on drug use among youth, Kandel (1978) concludes that sociodemographic variables have little predictive power for initiation into marijuana use. The national sample study mentioned earlier yielded similar findings: Demographic variables have minimal linkage to variation in problem drinking or marijuana involvement.

The point we draw from these observations is that the demographic environment is probably too conceptually distal from behavioral variation to be empirically useful. For environmental variables to be effective in social-psychological research, they need to be more proximal. If they are not variables that are perceived by the actor—the choice we made—they should probably represent the perceptions of others about aspects of the environment likely to be relevant to action.

Issues Related to Psychosocial Development

Several aspects of the developmental findings have implications that warrant discussion. First, the concept of transition proneness would appear to be useful in developmental research. Referring to a "readiness" to change status along a developmental continuum, its conceptual components are clear and their measurement is feasible. That it refers to a readiness to change *status* rather than to engage in a particular behavior needs emphasis; this was borne out by two aspects of the findings: that transition proneness was not behavior specific but implicated a set of transition-marking actions and that transition itself was associated with a constellation of personality changes, the kind of organized change that suggests a concomitant shift in self-identity. Although we have focused on transition initiated by engaging in transition-marking behaviors, it is also possible that transition proneness can be implemented by a cognitive reorganization of personality—a decision, for example, to be more independent or to become a more responsible person. Research on this latter aspect would indeed be illuminating.

Second, although the direction of developmental change in the High School Study was consistent whether the data were partitioned by sex, or grade, or even by time of onset of transition behavior, there was clear evidence in the trajectories of what has been called "cohort effects." This refers to the fact that the developmental curves for cohorts born in different years may differ in both level and shape. Because of our theoretical focus on the direction of change, we did not pursue an analysis of cohort effects, and in any case it is difficult to know how they might be interpreted. The argument that they reflect historical differences in life experience is not compelling when the interval between cohorts is only a year, rather than, say, a decade. An alternative possibility is that they simply reflect sampling variation, a possibility that might be ruled out in developmental studies by employing multiple samples in each birth cohort. Although they argue for the importance of dealing with cohort effects in their recent extensive review, Baltes, Cornelius, and Nesselroade (1978) concede finally that ". . . the available evidence on the role of cohort effects in behavioral development is largely descriptive; efforts at theoretical-explanatory analysis are rare and at best prototheoretical [p. 48]." Until work in this area is further advanced, not much more can be done with cohort effects than to acknowledge their existence and hope that that in itself will be heuristic.

One other aspect of the developmental findings was noteworthy; beginning to drink, more than marking a transition in status, seems to imply crossing a watershed. The pivotal character of becoming a drinker was evident in the fact that abstainers had remarkably low rates of engaging in any of the variety of problem behaviors assessed. Not using alcohol appears to be associated with an insulation against problem behavior that is also reflected in a distinctive pattern of conformity proneness in personality and the perceived environment. The interesting implication is that transition behaviors may be ontogenetically ordered, and the key developmental change may be the one involved in crossing the initial threshold—in this case, beginning to drink.

The Historical Specificity of the Findings

How much our findings are bounded by the period in which they were obtained and are specific to that point in history is interesting to contemplate. The interpretation we have made of particular behaviors, and the very notion of problem behavior, depend upon the social and personal meanings that are attached to them. Important changes have taken place in recent history, and their effects on those meanings may well be far reaching. The "hang-loose ethic" of the 1960s (see Simmons & Winograd, 1966, and Suchman, 1968) is no longer apposite as a summary of the orientation of youth, and Winick (1975) has catalogued a number of changes between the two decades, the 1960s and the 1970s. With regard to marijuana use and sexual activity, the shift in societal attitudes is unmistakable, and prevalence rates have increased markedly. Even legal policy toward marijuana use has undergone transformation, with decriminalization statutes in a number of places and a relaxation of enforcement elsewhere. Such changes are likely to change the meanings that have been associated with these behaviors.

In our own data, for example, there is evidence that traditional sex differences have begun to erode and that males and females are converging in their rates of involvement in problem behavior. The trend toward disappearance of greater conventionality among females is clearly apparent when the criterion is modest—any experience at all. When the criterion is more stringent—heavier involvement with marijuana or frequent drunkenness, for example—males still outdistance females. Whether the trend will continue as women's roles are redefined and sex-role distinctions diminish is difficult to anticipate, but if it does it will carry with it a secular change in the significance of female problem behavior. Similar secular change is likely in relation to age also, with a trend toward earlier onset and the dissipation of traditional age distinctions.

The implications of such changes seem to us more impactful on particular behaviors than on Problem Behavior Theory as a whole. Although specific behaviors may shift in their meaning and decay as appropriate criteria, the general processes and structures of the theory should retain a degree of invariance in relation to adolescent growth and development.

A Closing Remark

Beyond its aims to test a social-psychological theory and to advance knowledge about youth, the work we have reported has tried to place problem behavior in a perspective of normal development. Much of the behavior is problematic only in relation to age, and problem proneness can often mean no more than developmental precocity. This is not to minimize the seriousness of some of the behaviors, for example, the excessive use of alcohol. Our view is that a benign and regulated outcome is more likely if there is a societal effort to understand the processes that underlie the occurrence of such behavior. Repressive policies have been counterproductive, and interpretations of maladjustment appear to be efforts to divest society of its share of responsibility. It would be an important step forward for prevention and control if problem behavior in youth came to be seen as part of the dialectic of growth, a visible strand in the web of time.

References

Baltes, P. B., Cornelius, S. W., & Nesselroade, J. R. (1978). Cohort effects in behavioral development: Theoretical and methodological perspectives. In W. A. Collins (Ed.), *Minnesota symposia on child psychology* (Vol. 2, pp. 1–63). Hillsdale NJ: Lawrence Erlbaum Associates.

Block, J. (1971). *Lives through time*. Berkeley: Bancroft Books.

Braucht, G. N. (1974). A psychosocial typology of adolescent alcohol and drug users. In M. E. Chafetz (Ed.), *Alcoholism: A multilevel problem. Proceedings of the Third Annual Alcoholism Conference*. National Institute on Alcohol Abuse and Alcoholism (pp. 129–144). Washington, DC: U.S. Government Printing Office.

Chase, J. A., & Jessor, R. (1977). *A social-psychological analysis of marijuana involvement among a national sample of adolescents*. Unpublished report to National Institute on Alcohol Abuse and Alcoholism, Contract No. ADM 281-75-0028, January, pp. 1–99.

Donovan, J. E. (1977). A typological study of self-reported deviance in a national sample of adolescents. Unpublished doctoral dissertation, University of Colorado.

Donovan, J. E., & Jessor, R. (1976). *Problem drinking among adolescents: A social-psychological study of a national sample*. Unpublished report to National Institute on Alcohol Abuse and Alcoholism, Contract No. ADM 281-75-0028, July, pp. 1–116.

Elliott, D. S., & Voss, H. L. (1974). *Delinquency and dropout*. Lexington, MA: D. C. Heath.

Jessor, R., Graves, T. D., Hanson, R. C., & Jessor, S. L. (1968). *Society, personality, and deviant behavior: A study of a tri-ethnic community*. New York: Holt, Rinehart and Winston. (Reprinted by Krieger Publishing Co., 645 New York Ave., Huntington, NY, 1975.)

Jessor, R., & Jessor, S. L. (1973). The perceived environment in behavioral science: Some conceptual issues and some illustrative data. *American Behavioral Scientist, 16*, 801–828.

Jessor, R., & Jessor, S. L. (1978). Theory testing in longitudinal research on marijuana use. In D. B. Kandel (Ed.), *Longitudinal research on drug use: Empirical findings and methodological issues* (pp. 41–71). Washington, DC: Hemisphere (Wiley).

Kandel, D. B. (1978). Convergences in prospective longitudinal surveys of drug use in normal populations. In D. B. Kandel (Ed.), *Longitudinal research on drug use: Empirical findings and methodological issues* (pp. 3–38). Washington, DC: Hemisphere (Wiley).

Kenny, D. A. (1975). Cross-lagged panel correlation: A test for spuriousness. *Psychological Bulletin, 82*, 887–903.

Nesselroade, J. R., & Baltes, P. B. (1974). Adolescent personality development and historical change: 1970–1972. *Monographs of the Society for Research in Child Development* (Serial No. 154, Vol. 39, pp. 1–80).

Rachal, J. V., Williams, J. R., Brehm, M. L., Cavanaugh, B., Moore, R. P., & Eckerman, W. C. (1975). *A national study of adolescent drinking behavior, attitudes, and correlates*. (Prepared for National Institute on Alcohol Abuse and Alcoholism. Rep. No. PB-246-002; NIAAA/NCALI-75/27). Springfield, VA.: U.S. National Technical Information Service.

Sadava, S. W. (1973). Initiation to cannabis use: A longitudinal social psychological study of college freshmen. *Canadian Journal of Behavioral Science, 5*, 371–384.

Simmons, J. L., & Winograd, B. (1966). *It's happening: A portrait of the youth scene today*. Santa Barbara, CA: Marc-Laird Publications.

Suchman, E. A. (1968). The "hang-loose" ethic and the spirit of drug use. *Journal of Health and Social Behavior, 9*, 146–155.

Winick, C. (1975). Speculations on possible changes in youthful life-styles between the 1960's and 1970's. In D. J. Lettieri (Ed.), *Predicting adolescent drug abuse: A review of issues, methods and correlates* (National Institute on Drug Abuse Research Issue Series No. 11, pp. 55–60). Washington, DC: U.S. Government Printing Office.

Chapter 5
Problem Behavior Theory and the Transition to Young Adulthood

Richard Jessor, John Edward Donovan, and Frances Marie Costa

The primary aim of renewing and extending our longitudinal study of youth was to add to knowledge about psychosocial development beyond adolescence and, at the same time, to explore a portion of the life course—young adulthood—that was still largely uncharted. The research findings reported represent what we have been able to accomplish in pursuing that aim. Their significance, and the conclusions they support, are elaborated here.

The approach that was taken was guided by a conceptual framework—Problem Behavior Theory—that had proved useful earlier in achieving an understanding of problem behavior and psychosocial development in adolescence and youth. Whether its explanatory reach would include young adulthood as well was yet to be determined. Nevertheless, the domains of inquiry that were engaged—personality, the perceived environment, the social environment, behavior—and the key concepts that were measured—values, expectations, social and self attitudes, models for behavior—all derived from that theoretical perspective. The major theoretical formulation about the likelihood of occurrence of problem behavior was also retained: Psychosocial proneness to problem behavior in young adulthood was considered to be a resultant, reflecting the balance of instigations and controls in the various explanatory systems. And the theoretical posi-

Reprinted with permission from:
Jessor, R., Donovan, J. E., & Costa, F. M. (1991). Chapter 10: "Problem behavior and young adulthood: Continuities in change." In R. Jessor, J. E. Donovan & F. M. Costa, *Beyond adolescence: Problem behavior and young adult development* (pp. 273–295). New York: Cambridge University Press.

R. Jessor (✉)
Institute of Behavioral Science, University of Colorado at Boulder, Boulder, CO 80309, USA
e-mail: jessor@Colorado.edu

J.E. Donovan
University of Pittsburgh, School of Medicine, Pittsburgh, USA

F.M. Costa
University of Colorado Boulder, Boulder, CO 80309, USA

R. Jessor, *The Origins and Development of Problem Behavior Theory*,
Advancing Responsible Adolescent Development,
DOI 10.1007/978-3-319-40886-6_5

tion about psychosocial development as the outcome of person–environment interactions over time continued to shape the study and interpretation of developmental change.

Although the focus of the research was on a particular area of behavior—problem behavior—and on the utility of a particular theoretical formulation, the enterprise as a whole was also concerned with broader issues in behavioral science. Among those issues were how best to represent persons in research on social behavior, that is, what individual differences to measure; how to capture the environment as a source of variance in behavior, and the importance of distinguishing proximal from distal environments; the logic of person–environment interaction in both behavior and development; the organization and patterning of systems of social behavior; and the plasticity of development reflecting the contingencies of context and setting. In short, the pursuit of understanding about problem behavior was animated by the opportunity it provided to illuminate fundamental issues that transcend what might otherwise be a limited empirical focus.

The Stability of Change

With regard to one of those fundamental issues—the nature of psychosocial development—the weight of the evidence is quite clear: Despite substantial change between adolescence/youth and young adulthood, the developmental process is characterized by stability and continuity across those segments of the life course. This conclusion gains even greater significance, given that the two life stages tend to be markedly different in their social organization, their predominating roles, their life tasks, and their social norms, and that moving developmentally from the earlier to the later one entails major transitions for most young people, not only in daily activities and responsibilities but in social and self-definitions as well.

Stability and consistency of individual differences were apparent in all three of the major explanatory systems—personality, the perceived environment, and behavior—when examined directly by stability coefficients. Somewhat stronger for the College Study than the High School Study, and considerably stronger across the two-year interval within young adulthood than across the eight-/nine-year interval between adolescence/youth and young adulthood, the magnitude of the coefficients provides compelling support, overall, for a continuity perspective on psychosocial development. Of special interest is the somewhat greater stability of the personality system attributes compared with those in the other two explanatory systems. Consonant with the reports of others (Mortimer, Finch, & Kumka, 1982; Stein, Newcomb, & Bentler, 1986), the evident stability of personality attributes over this time period is one more refutation of the sterile controversy a decade ago about the very "existence" of personality and its enduringness.

Further support for developmental continuity was evident, at the system level, in the latent-variable analyses. Examining latent-variable measures of personality system proneness, perceived environment system proneness, and behavior system proneness between adolescence/youth and young adulthood, we found over-time correlations to be in the mid-.50s for the High School Study and in the mid-.60s for the College Study. Given the eight- or nine-year time interval and the major life changes involved, these are magnitudes that are, indeed, impressive.

In reviewing a large variety of studies of the development of personality *in* adulthood, their own included, McCrae and Costa (1990) report clear consensus on the repeated demonstrations of stability and consistency. And in a research effort more relevant to our own, on the development of attitudes, aspirations, self-concepts, and behaviors among young men between adolescence and adulthood, Bachman, O'Malley, and Johnston (1978) conclude: "The dominant picture that emerges from this research is not change but stability" (p. 221). Thus, our stability findings are in agreement with the work of others. Although important developmental change does occur, as we discuss in the next section, the research makes apparent that there is considerable stability and continuity in that change. It would be safe to conclude from our findings that the adolescent is parent of the young adult.

The Direction of Developmental Change: Toward an Increase in Psychosocial Conventionality

Within a developmental process characterized by stability, there is, of course, ample room for major change. Mean levels on the various attributes and characteristics being observed may increase or decrease with development, and all that stability implies is that the relative position of individuals in the distribution is conserved over the time interval: Those initially high on some characteristic—say, value on achievement—tend to remain high relative to the group; those initially low on some measure—say, on perceived friends models for deviance—tend to remain low relative to the group. Granted the evidence for stability, a major developmental question remains: Has there been significant psychosocial change between adolescence/youth and young adulthood, and, if so, what is its general nature?

As with the evidence on stability and consistency, the answer that emerges from the data is, again, quite clear. For our cohorts, psychosocial development beyond adolescence/youth was unmistakably in the direction of greater conventionality. This direction of change was apparent in all three explanatory systems; in each system, there was significant decline in problem behavior proneness, reflecting both a reduction in instigations and an increase in controls. The psychosocial "growth curves" illustrate change on some of the key theoretical variables: an increase in value on achievement, a decline in social criticism and alienation, an increase in attitudinal intolerance of deviance, and a decline in friends models for drug use (in the College Study only). This general direction of change—toward greater conventionality—between adolescence/youth and young adulthood not only was significant but in several instances also represented a complete reversal of the direction of developmental change *within* adolescence/youth, namely, toward *greater* problem behavior proneness or *un*conventionality.

The same direction of change toward conventionality was evident in the Behavior System as well, as indicated by the significant decline in self-reported general deviant behavior and declines in the proportion of problem drinkers and heavier marijuana users. The theoretical consonance of the decline in problem behavior with the parallel declines in problem behavior proneness in both the Personality System and the Perceived Environment System strengthens conviction about the developmental inference being drawn, that is, that there is an overall trend toward a reduction in problem behavior proneness and an increase in conventionality with development into young adulthood. Theoretical consonance was demonstrated in yet another way. It was demonstrated that those who showed a decrease in overall problem behavior between adolescence/youth and young adulthood showed an increase in psychosocial conventionality over that same time interval; those who showed an increase in problem behavior showed a decrease in conventionality; and those whose involvement in problem behavior did not change, did not change in conventionality either. These findings, at the group level, buttress the overall findings about the theoretical consonance of the developmental changes toward greater conventionality.

Although it is important to be able, empirically, to identify a major direction of developmental change associated with the passage into and through young adulthood, it would be mistaken to assume that all adolescents develop in the same way. Indeed, a particularly interesting contribution of this inquiry has been the demonstration of large individual differences in psychosocial development beyond adolescence. Partitioning the cohorts into groups that were High, Medium, or Low on conventionality (or problem behavior proneness) in adolescence/youth made it possible to reveal markedly different trajectories of development toward young adulthood for the three groups. Those who were initially high in conventionality showed little or no significant change between the two life stages on a number of key measures of problem behavior proneness; those, however, who were initially low in conventionality, that is, most unconventional, showed major change over time in the direction of greater conventionality; and those initially medium in conventionality fell in between, showing a medium amount of change toward conventionality. Where change occurred, then, it was toward increased conventionality for all three groups, but the amount of change and the rate of change yielded quite different developmental trajectories for the three groups. The similarity that all three groups show in level of conventionality by the time of reaching young adulthood belies the fact that *quite different paths were followed in getting there.* What is especially noteworthy in those findings is the evidence that the shift toward conventionality was most marked among those who were initially—in the early 1970s—the least conventional; by the early 1980s they had become much closer in conventionality to the other two groups, though still remaining less so as the stability findings would, of course, lead us to expect.

The developmental change toward a decline in problem behavior proneness or toward an increase in conventionality, while apparent in all three systems and on a variety of key theoretical attributes, was not without exception and qualification. Nevertheless, it is a directional change that is compatible with what is well-established in the literature about the developmental course of involvement in problem behavior. According to Gove (1985), "Virtually all forms of deviance that involve substantial risk and/or physically demanding behavior occur mainly among young persons, and the rates of such deviance decline sharply by the late twenties and early thirties" (p. 115). And a leading scholar reviewing this field states: "All common forms of deviance (drug use, theft, drinking, sexual promiscuity, fighting) seem to drop off with age" (Robins, 1980, p. 37).

The term "maturing out" has been applied to the diminution or abandonment of involvement in problem behavior that seems to occur in the mid- to late twenties, but what it really refers to, that is, what the underlying determinants of that process are, has not been well understood. Most often, the term is assumed to implicate the assumption of adult roles and exposure to the informal social controls they entail. Our own data did not permit us to examine this process directly, unfortunately. However, a recent secondary analysis of the data from the classical longitudinal study of delinquency by the Gluecks (1950, 1968) has reported compelling support for such an interpretation: "We have shown that job stability and marital attachment in adulthood are significantly related to changes in adult crime—the stronger the adult ties to work and family, the less crime and deviance among both [former] delinquents and controls" (Sampson & Laub, 1990, p. 625). And they add that change in young adulthood "appears to be systematically structured by adult bonds to social institutions" (p. 625).

This emphasis on the assumption of social roles and on the effects of their associated informal social controls is entirely consistent with the age-related drop off in problem behavior, and the Sampson and Laub findings are a welcome contribution to an understanding of the process of "maturing out." What our own findings add to such understanding is new evidence about the changes in personality and perceived environment attributes that are also associated with "maturing out," that is, with a decline in involvement in problem behavior. Whether the psychosocial changes at the individual level that we have identified and summarized as an increase in conventionality may, in fact, mediate between the assumption of adult roles and exposure to informal social controls, on the one hand, and the decline in problem behavior involvement, on the other hand, is certainly worthy of a future research effort.

Beyond support for stability and continuity in psychosocial development, then, the findings from this longitudinal study provide substantial evidence for developmental change. The overall trajectory of change, theoretically in the direction of greater conventionality and less involvement in problem behavior, has to be seen, however, as a composite of trajectories reflecting individual differences in amount, in direction, and in rate of change.

The Organization of Problem Behavior in Young Adulthood

The findings speak to another basic issue in behavioral science research, namely the degree to which there is organization, patterning, or structure in behavior in young adulthood. In the problem behavior field, the tradition has long been to specialize in one or another of its components—delinquency, drug use, drinking behavior, sexuality—and entire professional careers have been shaped by that tradition, as has also the organization of the research support bureaucracy in the various federal institutes. The alternative perspective places emphasis on the larger class to which, it can be argued, the various component behaviors all belong, namely, the category of normative transgression, or deviance, or, as we have referred to it throughout this book, problem behavior. The argument can be made that topographically different behaviors can serve the same purpose (e.g., the affirmation of peer group membership) and therefore can functionally substitute for one another. It can also be argued that the social ecology of problem behaviors is such that different problem behaviors—say, smoking and drinking, or drug use and crime, or alcohol use and aggression—are often learned together and expected to be performed together. Arguments such as these suggest that there should be organization or structure among the various problem behaviors and that they should show some degree of covariation. It was this kind of thinking that led to our formulation of behavior as a *system* in Problem Behavior Theory, and to our including in the system a structure of interrelated problem behaviors and a structure of conforming behaviors.

In our earlier work on adolescents, considerable attention was given to exploring the extent and degree of covariation that existed among the various measures of adolescent problem behavior. In light of the results of those explorations, it was proposed that problem behavior in adolescence might well constitute a *syndrome.* Since then, there has been substantial empirical support for that notion. Coming at the same basic issue from another perspective, Robins's conclusion from her review of longitudinal research on deviance is fully consonant with the connotations of the syndrome concept: "The best predictor of any later deviant act always seems to be earlier deviant behavior, and the specific *nature* of that earlier deviant behavior seems uniformly to be relatively unimportant" (1980, p. 36).

Having established earlier that the idea of covariation among problem behaviors and the syndrome concept were apposite to the adolescence/youth phase of this research, we undertook to examine the same issue in the young adult data. The key question was whether development beyond adolescence sustained the observed organization of problem behavior or, conceivably, resulted in its dissolution.

The findings from the bivariate correlational analyses, the categorical cross-tabulations, and the maximum-likelihood factor analysis were all convergent in showing interrelatedness among the five different young adult problem behaviors—frequency of drunkenness, frequency of marijuana use, other illicit drug use, general deviant behavior, and cigarette smoking—and in showing also that a single underlying factor could account for the observed correlations among those behaviors. In this respect, the young adult findings were similar to those for adolescence/youth, and they provided support for the idea of a syndrome of problem behavior in young adulthood.

It was possible to examine the issue in yet another way by establishing, for the first time, latent variables for each of the different problem behaviors, and then applying structural equation modeling techniques to their interrelations. The results of that approach were that a single second-order latent variable of behavior system proneness can account for the correlations among the five latent-variable measures of problem behavior. This structural modeling approach adds particularly compelling support for the idea of covariation among problem behaviors in young adulthood.

It seems clear, then, at least for our cohorts, that there is, indeed, organization and structure among a variety of problem behaviors in young adulthood, just as there was in adolescence/youth. The importance of such knowledge lies in the impetus it provides for researchers to seek understanding of behavioral *repertoires*, rather than continuing to focus on single behaviors alone. It lies also in the challenge it poses for intervention efforts to transcend a preoccupation with separate problem behaviors as if they existed in isolation from one another.

Explaining Young Adult Problem Behavior

The explanatory reach of Problem Behavior Theory as an account of variation in problem behavior in the later developmental stage of young adulthood—and in the historical era of the late 1970s and early 1980s—was not something that could simply be taken for granted. From a historical perspective alone, there had been major increases in the prevalence of certain problem behaviors—particularly illicit drug use and nonmarital sexual activity; normative orientations had been shifting toward greater acceptance, and social control responses were undergoing widespread modulation. From a developmental perspective, the constraints of age-graded norms and the idea of transition out of adolescence would no longer be apposite as explanatory formulations for problem behavior involvement. In addition, young adulthood entails exposure to very different institutional contexts—the family and work, for example, as contrasted with the school and peer group—and these settings provide different structures of opportunity, of norms, and of formal and informal controls. Whether a conceptual framework emphasizing personality and perceived environment variables that represented instigations to and controls against normative transgression among adolescents/youth in the early 1970s would retain its relevance for both a later developmental stage and a later historical era had to be treated, at the very least, as problematic. Efforts were made to enhance the age appropriateness of the item content of the measures, and to inquire about satisfactions and stress in the life areas of young adulthood, but the key variables remained those that had been relied on in the earlier phase of the longitudinal study.

The continuing relevance of the Problem Behavior Theory framework for young adulthood is one of the major conclusions to be drawn from this follow-up study. The cross-sectional multivariate analyses provide a substantial account of the variation in problem behavior involvement in young adulthood, one that holds for both genders, in both studies, and in both years—1979 and 1981—of the follow-up. A summary appraisal of the overall findings can best be gained by considering the multiple regressions of the composite measure of involvement in problem behavior, the Multiple Problem Behavior Index, on the combined theoretical systems—personality, perceived environment, and behavior. The 11 key measures used in the Overall Psychosocial Proneness regressions yielded multiple correlations of .76, .75, .77, and .63 for the High School Study men and women and the College Study men and women, respectively. Thus, for the first three groups, over 50 percent of the variance in young adult problem behavior in 1981 is accounted for by the theoretical framework, and it is close to 40 percent for the fourth group. This magnitude of the account of variance is quite robust across the 1979, Year V data set, as well, and it also compares very closely with that obtained in the 1972/73, Year IV, adolescence/youth data set, where the respective multiple correlations were .74, .77, .68, and .68.

When the theoretical framework is applied, separately, to the various component problem behaviors, the multiple correlations are similar for marijuana use, somewhat lower for frequency of drunkenness and for the use of other illicit drugs, somewhat lower still for general deviance, and lowest for cigarette smoking (on this latter measure, the multiple correlations fall short of statistical significance for the College Study men and women).

The young adult theoretical findings also parallel those from the adolescence/youth phase in the relative contribution made by the different explanatory systems. In general, the Perceived Environment System yields larger multiple correlations with the Multiple Problem Behavior Index (and with its various component behaviors) than does the Personality System. The reason for this, in the present data set, would seem to be the same one that applied in the 1972/73 data set: The key measures in the Perceived Environment System, especially Friends' Approval and Friends Models for Drug Use, are more proximal to problem behavior than are the measures in the Personality System. Where this is *not* the case—for example, for General Deviance—the Personality System includes the highly proximal (and parallel) measure of Attitudinal Intolerance of Deviance, and that is the reason why the Personality System now yields a larger multiple correlation than the Perceived Environment System. Another instance of such reversal of the contributions of the two systems occurs with regard to the conventional behavior of church attendance. The highly proximal measure of Religiosity is included in the Personality System, and that is what enables it to supervene the Perceived Environment System in amount of variance accounted for in Church Attendance. This general issue of the relative contribution of the two systems to explanation is important to clarify. Appropriate recognition of the role played by the proximal versus distal relation of a measure to a behavioral criterion can forestall inappropriate conclusions about whether it is personality or the environment that is more important in determining behavior. From an interactionist perspective, any such conclusion would be conceptually meaningless.

There is another issue, however, that *is* relevant to an interactionist perspective, and that pertains to the increase in the explanatory account that should occur when both the Personality System and the Perceived Environment System are considered *jointly*. In the multivariate, cross-sectional analyses of the Multiple Problem Behavior Index, when personality proneness and perceived environment proneness are combined into psychosocial proneness, there is, indeed, a significant increment in variance explained (R^2) over the variance explained by either system alone. This is generally the case for the separate criterion behaviors as well. Findings such as these parallel those from the adolescence/youth phase of the research as well, and they contribute new empirical support for the logic of the interactionist position in behavioral science research.

Although the magnitude of the explanatory account in young adulthood is very nearly identical to that in adolescence/youth, the pattern of variables playing a key role is somewhat different. At the young adult stage, the motivational-instigation variables are relatively less important (Value on and Expectation for Achievement) or unimportant (Value on and Expectation for Independence) compared with the role they played in the earlier phase of the research. Internal-External Locus of Control and Self-Esteem are only weakly or inconsistently related to problem behavior, but this was also the case in the earlier phase. And Alienation is more consistently related to problem behavior in young adulthood than it was in adolescence/youth. On the other hand, the similarity of the patterns is extensive; it includes the personal belief variable of Social Criticism, the personal control variables of Intolerance of Deviance and Religiosity, the proximal perceived environment variables of Friends'

Approval of and Friends Models for Problem Behavior, and the Behavior System measure of conventional behavior, Church Attendance. The pattern of explanatory variables in young adulthood, representing all three of the theoretical systems, constitutes what we have been referring to as "psychosocial conventionality," and, in this regard, it is almost isomorphic with the conventionality pattern that emerged from the adolescence/youth phase of the research.

The applicability and relevance of the Problem Behavior Theory framework for young adulthood suggest that there is a certain degree of developmental invariance in the explanation of problem behavior. In demonstrating explanatory invariance across the adolescent/youth and young adult life stages, the research extends the developmental generality of the theoretical framework. Kandel reached a similar conclusion for the specific behavior of marijuana use in her follow-up study of adolescents into young adulthood (to ages 24 and 25): "The social psychology of marijuana use is… much the same in young adulthood as in adolescence…. [M]arijuana involvement is associated with the same factors that had previously been reported for younger populations of junior high school, senior high school, and college students" (1984, p. 208). The evidence for developmental invariance in the explanatory account is complemented by evidence for a degree of historical invariance as well. In our own work over the years since the late 1960s, in both local and national samples (Donovan & Jessor, 1978; Jessor, Chase, & Donovan, 1980; Jessor, Donovan, & Widmer, 1980), very similar patterns of social and psychological variables have been found to be associated with adolescent problem behavior, and with remarkably similar magnitudes of association. And recently, in a new longitudinal study of over 2000 urban middle school and high school adolescents, we have again found the same pattern; the multiple correlations of overall psychosocial proneness with the Multiple Problem Behavior Index in the new (1989) data are .70, .74, .70, .71, for middle school males and females and high school males and females, respectively. Such evidence for both developmental and historical invariance in the explanation of problem behavior strengthens conviction about the utility of the theoretical framework.

One of the adaptations that was made to the framework, both to extend it and to examine an alternative formulation about the determinants of problem behavior, was the addition of the concept of stress to the young adult phase of the research. The mapping and measurement of stress were admittedly limited, and that, in turn, sharply limits the conclusions that can be drawn. What was found, nevertheless, was that measures of stress related in a modest way to the Multiple Problem Behavior Index, and to one of its components, General Deviance, except for the College Study men in both instances. The amount of variance accounted for by the two stress measures taken together reached, at best, 11 percent for the Index and 18 percent for the measure of General Deviance. What was most persuasive theoretically, however, was that the addition of the stress measures to the measures of overall psychosocial proneness added no new source of variance and did not increase the R^2 associated with the latter. On the basis of these results, it seems clear that the concept of stress, at least as measured, does not extend the reach of the larger theoretical framework, nor does it capture a unique source of variance that is not already mapped by the larger framework.

As a theory of the middle range, an explanatory formulation limited to the social and psychological factors that account for involvement in normative transgression, Problem Behavior Theory—in addition to its established relevance for adolescence/youth—can now be considered apposite to the developmental stage of young adulthood.

The Predictability of Problem Behavior in Young Adulthood

Conviction about the usefulness of the conceptual framework was strengthened by the results of the cross-sectional and the developmental analyses. Such conviction can be buttressed further, and in an especially compelling way, by a demonstration that the variables in the framework measured earlier, have *predictiveness*, over a significant time interval, for later involvement in problem behavior. The bivariate, multivariate, and structural equation modeling analyses were focused on just such a demonstration.

The results from the multiple regression analyses predicting variation in the 1981 Multiple Problem Behavior Index from overall psychosocial proneness measured in 1972/73 provide clear and consistent evidence of significant and—given the length of the time interval—substantial predictability. The multiple correlations for High School Study men and women and College Study men and women, respectively, are .52, .42, .66, and .59. Problem behavior proneness in each of the theoretical systems—personality, perceived environment, and behavior—in adolescence/youth is significantly associated with later variation in actual involvement in problem behavior in young adulthood. The results for the various component problem behaviors are generally similar, although weaker for general deviant behavior and for cigarette smoking.

In order to assess the predictability of young adult involvement in problem behavior in a way that would take account of the unreliability of measurement at both time points, and that would illuminate the pathways by which the adolescent/youth precursors were linked to young adult problem behavior, we employed structural equation modeling with latent variables. These analyses reveal substantial correlations between the latent variable for personality system proneness and for perceived environment system proneness in adolescence/youth, on the one hand, and the latent variable for the Behavior System in young adulthood, on the other. For the High School Study, these respective latent-variable correlations are .56 and .41; for the College Study, they are .75 and .55.

More interesting, perhaps, than the magnitude of the over time correlations between these latent variables are the "causal" pathways in the structural diagrams for both the High School Study and the College Study. The fact that is most salient is the key role of personality system proneness over the time interval. Personality system proneness in adolescence/youth has both direct and indirect linkages with the young adult behavior system latent variable in the High School Study, and a significant indirect path in the College Study. Neither the perceived environment system nor the behavior system latent variables in adolescence/youth show that extent of linkage over time. In providing a representation of "causal" structure, the structural model helps to illuminate what underlies the over-time correlations among the latent variables. The prime role of the Personality System, and of its stability, is noteworthy. The conventional wisdom in the field was cogently summarized by Robins as follows: "The best predictor of any later deviant act always seems to be earlier deviant behavior" (1980, p. 36). The present findings reopen that conclusion, and they raise an important question about the extent to which it may simply reflect the failure, in most investigations, to exhaust the causal contribution of other domains by more comprehensive and systematic measurement of *non*behavioral predictor variables.

That young adult involvement in problem behavior can be forecast by reliance on its theoretical precursors is another significant conclusion of this longitudinal study. The predictive findings not only strengthen the theory but also offer some potential for designing early intervention efforts on a more systematic basis than happens to be the usual practice.

Outcomes of Adolescent Involvement in Problem Behavior

Whether involvement in problem behavior in adolescence/youth creates a legacy for later life was another developmental issue that our longitudinal inquiry was able to address. The results of several types of analysis—analysis of variance, multiple regression, and structural equation modeling—were convergent in their support for two major conclusions. The first conclusion is that there is significant continuity in involvement in problem behavior across the two life stages for our cohorts; the greater the involvement in problem behavior in adolescence/youth, the greater the involvement in problem behavior in young adulthood. Our findings in this regard are entirely consistent with other research that has followed young people beyond adolescence.

The second conclusion, supported equally strongly by the analyses, is that involvement in problem behavior in adolescence/youth does *not* implicate variation in *other* outcomes in young adulthood—outcomes that range across status attainment, work, family, friendship, health, self-esteem, alienation, political participation, and overall life satisfaction. None of the results suggests that there is a "spillover" from the problem behavior area to these other life outcomes, or that adolescent involvement in problem behavior has compromised later development or has mortgaged the future for the youth in our research. This second conclusion will be somewhat more controversial with respect to the literature, and it warrants further attention. Some of the literature is quite compatible with this conclusion—for example, the reports by Power and Estaugh (1990) and by Newcomb and Bentler (1987, 1988). But Newcomb and Bentler (1988) do raise some differences in outcomes (they term them "consequences") in at least some areas of young adult life, such as marital and job instability, related to variation in earlier involvement in the specific behavior of drug use. Kandel and colleagues (1986), following up the later outcomes of earlier adolescent drug involvement, also report young adult variation in regard to work and marital stability (although the unique effects of adolescent drug use disappear when use *between* adolescence and young adulthood is controlled for).

And in their secondary analysis of the Gluecks' delinquency data, Sampson and Laub (1990) state: "Childhood antisocial behaviors are also predictive of economic, family, educational, and employment problems up to eighteen years later," and they call attention to "the generality of the link between childhood delinquency and troublesome adult behavior" (p. 616).

Perhaps the most important fact to raise in attempting to reconcile discrepancies between our findings and those of others is that our research was based upon normal samples of youth drawn from school-based populations rather than from treatment centers or penal institutions. Thus, the seriousness of and committedness to problem behavior in adolescence/youth was likely to be less than that in samples of the latter sort. In the Gluecks' data, for example, the delinquent sample had a persistent record of adjudicated delinquency, with an average of 3.5 *convictions*, and had been committed to correctional school in Massachusetts (see also Farrington & West, 1990). The relevance of this issue of seriousness of involvement in problem behavior in adolescence is raised in another way by Newcomb and Bentler (1989) who, after stating that "all drug *abuse* is destructive and can have devastating consequences" (p. 247; italics added), go on to say that "infrequent, intermittent, or occasional use of drugs by a basically healthy teenager probably has few short-term and no long-term negative or adverse consequences" (pp. 247–248). Although the analyses we made of "heavier" marijuana use in adolescence yielded findings that were not different from those for problem behavior as a whole, and although "heavier" use in our study did mean regular use, that is, at least two or three times a week, still, even that level of involvement is simply not as serious or committed as, for example, a "daily use" criterion would connote.

The second most important fact to raise is that our research engaged youth who were largely middle-class in socioeconomic status and who had considerable access to opportunity. Their general wellbeing as young adults was apparent from the qualitative descriptions presented earlier. By contrast, Sampson and Laub describe the Gluecks' youth as boys who "grew up in high-risk environments characterized by poverty, social disorganization, and exposure to delinquency and antisocial conduct" (1990, p. 612). An interactionist position about development would consider that later-life outcomes of adolescent involvement in problem behavior would be contingent on the nature of the contexts in which later development takes place. Contexts of poverty and social disorganization are obviously less likely than middle-class contexts to provide resources for overcoming a history of problem behavior, or to make "second chances" available, that is, to be "forgiving" in the sense of maintaining open opportunity despite previous problem behavior involvement.

A third fact is age. The differential consequences of adolescent drug use that are described by Newcomb and Bentler (1988) refer to young adults with a mean age of just under 22 years (range, 21–23). This is, if anything, very young adulthood and, indeed, an age that we have characterized as "youth" rather than young adulthood. Such an early age of follow-up may yield differences that could well disappear with further development into young adulthood, that is, into the latter part of the third decade of life where our own follow-up took place. The issue of age is potentially important in another way. Although we found no differences in a wide variety of young adult life areas that were related to variation in earlier involvement in problem behavior, the possibility remains that differences will yet emerge with later development into adulthood and midlife. What makes that more than just a logical possibility is the fact that those who were more involved in problem behavior in adolescence/youth were also shown to be more involved in problem behavior in young adulthood. It is that greater young adult involvement that could, perhaps, reverberate into other life areas as development begins to traverse the fourth decade of life.

These issues and, of course, other kinds of sample differences may be relevant to the differences in findings that have emerged from the different studies. Nevertheless, it is important to emphasize that there is still considerable consonance between our findings and those of others, and that the present findings are coherent across different adolescent/youth problem behaviors and for a wide variety of young adult outcomes. For largely middle-class cohorts such as ours, growing beyond adolescence in the 1970s in the United States, early problem behavior involvement does not seem to mortgage the future—at least through young adulthood.

The Limits of Inference

Whatever the compellingness and coherence of a set of findings, no inquiry—much less one that deals with complex human experience and behavior extended in time—can sustain inferences that are without some degree of ambiguity. That is to say, all scientific inference—even that drawn from exquisitely controlled laboratory experiments—is vulnerable to plausible alternative inferences being drawn from the same set of observations. The quest in every scientific investigation, and the very raison d'être of research design, is the reduction of ambiguity of inference (see Jessor, Graves, Hanson, & Jessor, 1968, Chap. 4). In contemporary field studies, efforts to reduce the ambiguity of inference involve, increasingly, the collection of observations from different sources, with different methods, and in different contexts, in order to permit "triangulation" or convergence on the sought-after conclusions. This orientation to inquiry has been generalized under the rubric of "multiplism" in a seminal essay by Cook (1985) in which he argues for an approach to knowledge growth based upon a "critical multiplism." The latter entails multiple measures of a construct, multiple methods, multiple studies, multiple (i.e., rival) models and hypotheses, multiple analytic approaches, multiple populations, etc., along with an unremitting concern for eliminating bias (a chronic alternative inference) from knowledge generation.

The multiplist orientation is a useful frame of reference for considering the limitations, as well as the advantages, of our Young Adult Follow-Up Study. Its initial limitation was, of course, the sample drawn at the outset in 1969 for the High School Study and in 1970 for the College Study. Both samples had less than desirable initial participation rates. Although subsequent attrition was modest, and although retention beyond the adolescence/youth phase was quite remarkable, nevertheless, this constitutes a potential source of bias (i.e., an alternative inference) that needs to be acknowledged. We spent time in the earlier book (Jessor & Jessor, 1977) and now in this volume stressing the coherence and the robustness of our findings, as well as their replication in multiple studies by us and by others. Persuasive as those arguments may be, this limitation, unfortunately, remains.

A second limitation pertains to the racial/ethnic and socioeconomic homogeneity of the research samples. As we noted earlier, there is the possibility that particular findings might have been different had there been representation of other ethnic and social class groups in the samples whose lives we have followed. Clearly, multiple populations would have enhanced a claim for generality of inference. A third important limitation is the relative absence of participants who showed extreme involvement in problem behavior, an absence largely due to drawing normal samples from the schools and the university in a middle-class community. Although a substantial range of variation in problem behavior involvement did obtain, the distribution was doubtless truncated at its extreme tail.

The next limitation pertains to the key method employed in the research. The reliance on self-report throughout the research, in both its earlier and its later phases, means that multiple methods were not engaged, and this is the fourth important limitation. Whether or not the other methods would have been feasible in this inquiry is another question; the fact remains that the findings are tied to a single method rather than representing the convergence of multiple methods. Further, the reliance on a questionnaire as a single information source that included measures of all the variables of interest, can constitute what Cook refers to as a source of constant bias. Fortunately, on this issue, measurement was automatically made "heterogeneous" whenever we undertook time-extended analyses. In the descriptive analyses, the predictive analyses, and the outcome analyses, the data being linked came from *different* questionnaires, questionnaires that were separated in time by as much as eight or nine years. In such instances, common method variance as a source of constant bias is no longer a reasonable alternative inference.

The fifth and final limitation has to do with the research design, itself, more particularly, with the long time interval between adolescence/youth and young adulthood in which no measurement was made. The result is that inferences drawn *across* that time period—for example, the information in the growth curves—can well be misleading in failing to represent changes in the trajectories that could possibly have occurred *within* that interval. All sorts of ups and downs rather than a smooth line may, in fact, have characterized the interim period between adolescence/youth and young adulthood. Multiple data points within the follow-up interval beyond adolescence would have been preferable, instead of just the two in 1979 and 1981. Happily, there was, at least, more than one!

Several positive features of the research enterprise balance these limitations. Most important, perhaps, has been our reliance on the same theoretical formulation that had proved useful in a variety of studies in a variety of contexts over a period of decades. This feature represents what might well be termed "cumulative multiplism." In addition, in the present study, there were multiple samples, multiple measures of the same construct, and multiple, even if sometimes redundant, analytic methods; in short, the general orientation of multiplism was, indeed, well represented in the Young Adult Follow-Up Study.

Further, the research findings were always examined separately in the four groups—the High School Study men and women and the College Study men and women. Neither gender differences nor study differences emerged as important or consistent in the analyses, and therefore, the generality of findings across the four subsamples became a criterion for conviction about a particular relationship. Although conservative, this approach constituted another implementation of the multiplist orientation.

Two additional points are worth noting. First, when personality concepts are employed in social research, they usually have their origin in psychopathology or clinical theory. Thus, the different formulation employed in this research made the concept of personality and its measurement heterogeneous. The present conceptualization is at the sociocognitive level, a concept of personality that includes values, and attitudes, and self-definitions that reflect social experience, on the one hand, and that can link logically to social behavior, on the other. The value of this kind of representation of the person, and the value of the particular variables that were assessed, are quite evident from the overall findings and, especially, from the key role that was played by the personality system in mediating the predictive relationships between adolescence/youth and young adulthood. The summary dimension of conventionality-unconventionality, a key aspect of the social personality concept, should certainly engage the interest of personality researchers in their future work on social behavior.

Second, the effectiveness of the theoretical formulation in accounting for *conforming* behavior warrants mention. The multivariate explanation of church attendance, for example, accounts for over 60 percent of its variance in young adulthood, and the prediction of young adult educational attainment was also successful, based largely on adolescent measures of expectation for academic achievement and of academic performance. Concern with conventional behavior makes the research criterion heterogeneous. To that extent, it is another basis for conviction about the usefulness of Problem Behavior Theory.

A Final Word

We conclude this report with the sense of having added an increment to knowledge about young adulthood and about psychosocial development between adolescence and young adulthood. In our view, an increase in understanding of problem behavior beyond adolescence has also been achieved. The findings presented have a coherence and a consistency that, we believe, is compelling, and their theoretical relevance helps to amplify their significance.

The journey from the inception of this work, in 1969, has been a long one. As it comes to a close, we are reminded of the remarks of another scholar with the temerity to pursue complex longitudinal social research. He begins with the recognition that "research which tries to understand human experience within the time dimension is entering difficult and uncomfortable territory" (Edwards, 1989, p. 18). Nevertheless, such research is done, he goes on to tell us, "because of a belief that the years have more to teach about the human condition than can ever be learnt from one mere transient encounter with subject or sample." To this we would want to add only our own affirmation of assent.

References

Bachman, J. G., O'Malley, P. M., & Johnston, J. (1978). *Adolescence to adulthood: Change and stability in the lives of young men*. Ann Arbor: Institute for Social Research, University of Michigan.

Cook, T. D. (1985). Postpositivist critical multiplism. In R. L. Shotland & M. M. Mark (Eds.), *Social science and social policy* (pp. 21–62). Beverly Hills, CA: Sage.

Donovan, J. E., & Jessor, R. (1978). Adolescent problem drinking: Psychosocial correlates in a national sample study. *Journal of Studies on Alcohol, 39*, 1506–1524.

Edwards, G. (1989). As the years go rolling by: Drinking problems in the time dimension. *British Journal of Psychiatry, 154*, 18–26.

Farrington, D. P., & West, D. J. (1990). The Cambridge study in delinquent development: A long-term follow-up of 411 London males. In H. J. Kerner & G. Kaiser (Eds.), *Criminality: Personality, behavior and life history* (pp. 115–138). Berlin: Springer Verlag.

Glueck, S., & Glueck, E. (1950). *Unravelling juvenile delinquency*. New York: Commonwealth Fund.

Glueck, S., & Glueck, E. (1968). *Delinquents and nondelinquents in perspective*. Cambridge, MA: Harvard University Press.

Gove, W. R. (1985). The effect of age and gender on deviant behavior: A biopsychosocial perspective. In A. S. Rossi (Ed.), *Gender and the life course* (pp. 115–144). New York: Aldine.

Jessor, R., Chase, J. A., & Donovan, J. E. (1980). Psychosocial correlates of marijuana use and problem drinking in a national sample of adolescents. *American Journal of Public Health, 70*, 604–613.

Jessor, R., Donovan, J. E., & Widmer, K. (1980). *Psychosocial factors in adolescent alcohol and drug use: The 1978 National Study, and the 1974–78 Panel Study. Final report to Research Triangle Institute*. Boulder: Institute of Behavioral Science, University of Colorado.

Jessor, R., Graves, T. D., Hanson, R. C., & Jessor, S. L. (1968). *Society, personality, and deviant behavior: A study of a tri-ethnic community*. New York: Holt, Rinehart, & Winston.

Jessor, R., & Jessor, S. L. (1977). *Problem behavior and psychosocial development: A longitudinal study of youth*. New York: Academic Press.

Kandel, D. B. (1984). Marijuana users in young adulthood. *Archives of General Psychiatry, 41*, 200–209.

Kandel, D. B., Davies, M., Karus, D., & Yamaguchi, K. (1986). The consequences in young adulthood of adolescent drug involvement. *Archives of General Psychiatry, 43*, 746–754.

McCrae, R. R., & Costa, P. T., Jr. (1990). *Personality in adulthood*. New York: Guilford.

Mortimer, J. T., Finch, M. D., & Kumka, D. (1982). Persistence and change in development: The multi-dimensional self-concept. *Life-Span Development and Behavior, 4*, 263–313.

Newcomb, M. D., & Bentler, P. M. (1987). The impact of late adolescent substance use on young adult health status and utilization of health services: A structural equation model over four years. *Social Science and Medicine, 24*, 71–82.

Newcomb, M. D., & Bentler, P. M. (1988). *Consequences of adolescent drug use: Impact on the lives of young adults*. Newbury Park, CA: Sage.

Newcomb, M. D., & Bentler, P. M. (1989). Substance use and abuse among children and teenagers. *American Psychologist, 44*, 242–248.

Power, C., & Estaugh, V. (1990). Employment and drinking in early adulthood: A longitudinal perspective. *British Journal of Addiction, 85*, 487–494.

Robins, L. (1980). Alcoholism and labelling theory. In W. Gove (Ed.), *The labelling of deviance* (2nd ed., pp. 35–47). Beverly Hills, CA: Sage.

Sampson, R. J., & Laub, J. H. (1990). Crime and deviance over the life course: The salience of adult social bonds. *American Sociological Review, 55*, 609–627.

Stein, J. A., Newcomb, M. D., & Bentler, P. M. (1986). Stability and change in personality: A longitudinal study from early adolescence to young adulthood. *Journal of Research in Personality, 20*, 276–291.

Chapter 6
Problem Behavior Theory and the Problem Behavior Syndrome

John E. Donovan and Richard Jessor

The primary concern of the present studies was the structure or organization of the interrelations among various self-reported adolescent problem behaviors such as illicit drug use, problem drinking, delinquent behavior, and precocious sexual intercourse. The present studies also explored the generality of the syndrome of problem behavior that was found.

Problem behavior has been defined as "behavior that is socially defined as a problem, a source of concern, or as undesirable by the norms of conventional society . . . and its occurrence usually elicits some kind of social control response" (Jessor & Jessor, 1977, p. 33). According to this definition, a variety of different adolescent behaviors can be considered problem behaviors, including alcohol use, cigarette smoking, marijuana use, use of other illicit drugs, delinquent behavior, and precocious sexual intercourse.

There is considerable evidence that all of these different behaviors are associated in samples of adolescents from the normal population. The relations among these behaviors have been replicated in several independent nationwide samples of American adolescents as well as in numerous local community surveys, using a

---

Reprinted with permission from:
Donovan, J. E., & Jessor, R. (1985). Structure of problem behavior in adolescence and young adulthood. *Journal of Consulting and Clinical Psychology, 53*(6), 890–904.

J.E. Donovan,
University of Pittsburgh, School of Medicine, Pittsburgh, USA

R. Jessor (✉)
Institute of Behavioral Science, University of Colorado at Boulder, Boulder, CO, USA
e-mail: jessor@Colorado.edu

R. Jessor, *The Origins and Development of Problem Behavior Theory*,
Advancing Responsible Adolescent Development,
DOI 10.1007/978-3-319-40886-6_6

variety of self-report measures.[1] Most of these studies have examined only the bivariate relations among these behaviors, however, so little is actually known concerning the structure or organization underlying the obtained correlations.

The Jessor and Jessor research on Problem Behavior Theory (1977) suggested that drinking, problem drinking, marijuana use, delinquent behavior, and sexual intercourse may well constitute a "syndrome" of problem behavior in adolescence. Support for this syndrome notion emerged from the Jessors' analyses of data from two parallel longitudinal studies: one of junior high school students and one of college students. First, all of the problem behaviors were found to be positively associated in both samples; second, a composite index of multiple problem behaviors, encompassing all of the behaviors, correlated in the negative direction with measures of conforming or conventional behaviors, such as attendance at religious services and school performance; and third, the various problem behaviors correlated in a similar fashion with a number of personality and social environment variables that reflect unconventionality in the social-psychological framework of Problem Behavior Theory (Jessor & Jessor, 1977).

On the basis of these findings, it was suggested that the relations among the various problem behaviors were due to an underlying construct or latent variable of unconventionality in adolescence. Thus far, however, no analytic technique more rigorous than bivariate correlation has been used to test this proposition. The primary aim of the present studies, then, was to reanalyze the Jessor and Jessor (1977) data from their samples of high school and college-age youth to test more conclusively than before the hypothesis that the various problem behaviors reflect a single underlying common factor. To the extent that maximum likelihood factor analytic

---

[1] Alcohol use, cigarette smoking, marijuana use, and the use of other illicit drugs have been shown to be correlated among adolescents; that is, teenagers who are heavily involved with one of these drugs tend to be involved with others as well (Bachman, O'Malley, & Johnston, 1980; Block & Goodman, 1978; Hindelang, 1971; Huba, Wingard, & Bentler 1981; Hundleby, 1979; Istvan & Matarazzo, 1984; Jessor, Donovan, & Widmer, 1980; Jessor & Jessor, 1977; Johnson, 1973; Johnston, 1973; Miller et al., 1983; Single, Kandel, & Faust, 1974; Weitman, Scheble, Johnson, & Abbey, 1972; Zucker & Barron, 1973; Zucker & Devoe, 1975).

Marijuana use and other illicit drug use have also been found to correlate with problem drinking, a particular pattern of alcohol use that is characterized by frequent drunkenness and negative personal and social consequences (Donovan & Jessor, 1978; Jessor, Chase, & Donovan, 1980; Jessor, Donovan, & Widmer, 1980; Jessor & Jessor, 1977; Prendergast & Schaefer, 1974; Wechsler, 1976; Wechsler & Thum, 1973; Zucker & Barron, 1973; Zucker & Devoe, 1975).

Alcohol use, problem drinking, cigarette smoking, and illicit drug use also correlate with involvement in self-reported delinquent behavior (Donovan & Jessor, 1978; Hindelang, 1971; Hitachi 1969; Hundleby, 1979; Jessor, Donovan, & Widmer, 1980; Jessor & Jessor, 1977; Zucker & Barron, 1973; Zucker & Devoe, 1975) and with precocious involvement in sexual intercourse (Hundleby, 1979; Jessor & Jessor, 1977; Zucker & Barron, 1973; Zucker & Devoe, 1975).

Only a few of the studies have been concerned with the structure underlying the observed correlations. Their attention has been limited, however, to alcohol and drug use behavior (Hays, Widaman, DiMatteo, & Stacy, 1987; Huba, 1983; Huba & Bentler, 1979, 1982; Huba, Wingard, & Bentler, 1981). Delinquent or deviant behavior and precocious sexual intercourse have not been included in those analyses.

methods confirm that the relations among diverse problem behaviors do indeed reflect a single common factor, this would provide more compelling support for the notion of a syndrome of problem behavior in adolescence.

Beyond this primary objective were two further objectives for the present investigation. The second objective was to determine the generality of the factor-analytic results across adolescent samples. It is conceivable that the factor structure characterizing the problem behaviors may be specific to the Jessors' largely middle-class Anglo sample. The generality of this single-factor model, therefore, was tested using data collected on a more heterogeneous sample of adolescents by the Research Triangle Institute as part of the 1978 National Study of Adolescent Drinking (Rachal et al., 1980). Previous analyses of these data (Jessor, Donovan, & Widmer, 1980) supported the bivariate findings reported earlier by Jessor and Jessor (1977).

The third objective of the present studies was to determine whether the syndrome notion has developmental generality and can be demonstrated in data from young adults. Relatively little research has focused on problem behavior at this older age level, and even less research has investigated the relations among more than two or three problem behaviors (e.g., Bachman, O'Malley, & Johnston, 1984; Gove, Geerken, & Hughes, 1979; Kandel, 1984; Mechanic & Cleary, 1980; O'Donnell, Voss, Clayton, Slatin, & Room, 1976). In the present examination of the underlying structure of relations among various problem behaviors in young adulthood, we analyzed data collected as part of a follow-up study of the high school and college-age samples who had previously participated in the Jessors' study as adolescents or youth (Donovan, Jessor, & Jessor, 1983; Jessor, 1983; Jessor, Costa, Jessor, & Donovan, 1983; Jessor & Jessor, 1984).

Study I

The primary aim of this investigation—to determine whether diverse problem behaviors constitute a syndrome among the adolescents and college-age youth in the Jessor and Jessor (1977) data—was addressed in Study I.

Method

Because both the adolescent data dealt with in Study I and the young adult data addressed in Study III derived from the same larger study, the overall design of that study is presented briefly here.

Overall design of the Jessors' longitudinal study. The larger study was a six-wave, longitudinal study of psychosocial development that followed two parallel panel samples from adolescence through young adulthood. The high school sample consisted of 384 young adults (163 men, 222 women) who had participated in all six waves of data collection from junior high school through young adulthood.

These participants were initially selected in 1969 as part of a random sample of 1126 students stratified by sex and grade who were drawn from three junior high schools in a single school district in a small city in Colorado. Of the 1126 students initially sampled, 589 (53 %) participated with parental permission in the first of four annual data collection waves, A total of 432 of them (188 men, 244 women) completed all four annual questionnaires between 1969, when they were in Grades 7 through 9, and 1972, when they were in Grades 10 through 12.[2] These 432 young people were recontacted in 1979, when they were between 23 and 25 years old, and were asked to resume participation in the study; 403 of them (94 %) returned completed questionnaires. In 1981, 384 of these young adults participated in the sixth wave of data collection, when they were between 25 and 27 years old.

The parallel college sample consisted of 184 young adults (84 men, 100 women) who had participated in all six waves of data collection from freshman year of college through age 30. These participants were initially selected in 1970 as part of a random sample of freshman students in the College of Arts and Sciences of a large university in the same city. Of the 462 students initially contacted, 276 (approximately 60 %) completed questionnaires in the spring of 1970, and a total of 205 (92 men, 113 women) participated in all four annual waves of data collection (1970 through 1973).[3] In 1979, the 205 former participants, then approximately 28 years old, were recontacted, and 192 of them (94.1 %) returned completed questionnaires. In 1981, 184 of these young adults participated in the sixth wave of data collection, when they were around 30 years old.

Behavior measures. The questionnaires administered in all six data collections were about 50 pages long and consisted of a set of psychometric instruments developed to measure the personality, perceived environment, and behavior variables of Problem Behavior Theory (Jessor & Jessor, 1977). The measures of the behavior variables, all self-report, were generally very similar for both the high school and college sample questionnaires in all years.

The following problem behavior measures were examined in the data from the high school or college years: Times Drunk in the Past Year, a measure of the frequency with which a respondent had been drunk or "very, very high" on alcohol in

[2] In 1972, the fourth year of testing, 483 students completed questionnaires. This group comprised 82 % of the sample who participated in the first year of the study. Of these 483, 432 had taken the annual questionnaires in all 4 years. Comparisons on a variety of personality, social environment, and behavior measures assessed in 1969 showed that these 432 students were not different on most measures from those who participated in the research for fewer than 4 years (see Jessor & Jessor, 1977, pp. 46-47).

[3] A total of 226 young people participated in the fourth year of testing in 1973, when they were either seniors, transfer students, graduates, or college drop-outs. This group comprised 82 % of those who took the questionnaire in the first year of the study. Of these 226, 205 had completed all four annual questionnaires. Comparisons between this 4-year sample and those who participated only 1 or 2 years demonstrated that there were no real differences in conventionality between these groups in the 1970 data (see Jessor & Jessor, 1977, p. 51).

the past year, was used to represent problem drinking (range, 0–99)[4]; Frequency of Marijuana Use in the Past Six Months assessed how often a respondent had used marijuana or hashish in the designated time interval (range, 0–99); Frequency of Sexual Experience measured how often a respondent had engaged in sexual intercourse ("ever" for the high school sample; "in past year" for the college sample); General Deviant Behavior in the Past Year is a 26-item summative scale assessing how frequently in the past year a respondent had engaged in socially disapproved behaviors including shoplifting, vandalism, lying, truancy, fighting, parental defiance, and other behavior (range, 0–104; $\alpha=.8$).[5] For the most part, the measures focus on recent patterns of behavior rather than on "ever" experience.[6]

Conforming or conventional behavior was also included in certain of the analyses to provide a general test of the discriminant validity of the problem behavior measures and to serve as an anchor in the interpretation of the underlying common factor. Conventional behavior was represented in these analyses by the following two measures: Church Attendance Frequency in the Past Year, a measure of the number of times respondents attended religious services (range, 0–99); and School Performance, a self-report of grade point average (GPA; 0.0 to 4.0) for the previous semester (fall). These two conventional behavior measures were the only ones included in these analyses because they were the only measures in the category that were assessed in all of the high school and college questionnaires. The self-report measure of GPA was found to correlate .8 with GPA as recorded in school records. The four problem and two conventional behavior measures are described further in the Jessor and Jessor (1977) study.

Data analysis strategy. In both the adolescent and college data, the analyses were carried out separately on data from the third and fourth waves of data (referred to as Year 3 and Year 4, respectively) for each of four Sex by Sample groups (high school men and women and college men and women). Within each sample, the factor analyses were first carried out on the Year 4 data (1972 for the high school sample, 1973 for the college sample) and then replicated using the Year 3 data (1971 for the high school sample, 1972 for the college sample). Members of the youngest grade-cohort in the high school sample (60 men, 81 women) were dropped from the analyses because they had not been asked about sexual intercourse in Year 3. This is also the

[4] For these analyses, scores on the Times Drunk in the Past Year measure were recoded from blank to zero for abstainers and noncurrent drinkers. A similar strategy was also used for reported frequency of marijuana use. Adolescents who had never used marijuana or hashish or who had not used it in the past 6 months received scores of zero on the measure rather than a blank.

[5] The variety of behaviors in the General Deviant Behavior scale were dealt with as a summative scale rather than as separate items in the factor analyses because of the greater reliability of the scale and the restricted variances on the individual behavior items.

[6] Some of the behaviors occur so infrequently for most adolescents that standard short-term recall periods would result in scores with very low means. For this reason, Frequency of Marijuana Use asks about a shorter time period than do Times Drunk and General Deviant Behavior. The question on sexual intercourse was limited to reports of ever experiencing it because of the sensitivity of this question for the high school population.

reason why our factor analyses excluded the first and second waves of data. The factor analyses for the high school sample were therefore based on data from 102 men and 142 women; the factor analyses for the college sample were based on data from 84 men and 100 women.

In each factor analysis, the hypothesis was tested that a single common factor can account for the correlations among the problem behaviors. Basically, this was determined through a comparison of the observed correlations among the behaviors with the correlations among the behaviors predicted from the one-factor model. If the one-factor model were correct, the observed correlation between any two behaviors in the matrix would be equal to the product of these behaviors' estimated loadings on the common factor. The Jöreskog factor analysis procedure, available as part of the Statistical Package for the Social Sciences, Version 8.3 (Nie, Hull, Jenkins, Steinbrenner, & Bent, 1975), was used to compute a large-sample chi-square test of the discrepancy between the two matrices of observed and predicted correlations among the behaviors. A nonsignificant ($p>.05$) chi-square value would provide evidence in support of the hypothesis of a single common factor; a significant chi-square value would suggest that more than one common factor underlies the behaviors.

Results

The Pearson correlations on which the factor analyses were based are presented in Table 6.1 for the high school men and women and for the college men and women. For the high school sample, in both the Year 4 (1972) and Year 3 (1971) data, the correlations among all four measures of problem behavior—Times Drunk, Frequency of Marijuana Use, Frequency of Sexual Experience, and General Deviant Behavior—were statistically significant except for two correlations in the Year 4 data for women. The correlations between the problem behavior measures and the measures of conventional behavior were generally in the negative direction, as predicted, but were neither sizable nor consistent. For the college sample data, the correlations among the behavior measures were not as large or as consistent as those observed for the younger high school sample. In the Year 3 data, the correlations among the problem behaviors were more similar to the Year 4 correlations for the high school sample than were the correlations for the college sample in the Year 4 data. Overall, the correlations in the eight adolescent data matrices presented in Table 6.1 were adequate for the proposed maximum likelihood factor analyses, given that application of Bartlett's test of sphericity (Bartlett, 1950) to each of these matrices resulted in a significant chi-square value ($p<.01$) in all cases.

Maximum likelihood tests for one common factor. Table 6.2 presents the results of the factor analyses. All four of the chi-square tests on the Year 4 data demonstrated that only a single common factor was needed to account for the correlations among the problem behaviors. There were no statistically significant discrepancies ($p<.05$) between the observed correlation matrices and the matrices of correlations derived from the one-factor model. In all cases, the problem behaviors loaded positively on the underlying common factor, and all but one of the loadings—for Frequency of

Table 6.1 Correlations among selected measures of problem and conventional behavior in years 4 and 3 by sex and sample in each year

	High school men\women[a]						College men\women[b]					
Measure	1	2	3	4	5	6	1	2	3	4	5	6
Year 4												
Problem Behavior												
1. Times Drunk in the Past Year		.07	.23***	.23***	–.04	–.02		.12	.19*	.17*	–.13	–.18*
2. Frequency of Marijuana Use in the Past 6 Months	.25**		.12	.29†	–.24***	.09	.26**		.35†	.07	–.20**	–.26***
3. Frequency of Sexual Experience	.24**	.25***		.41†	–.18**	–.04	.03	–.11		.19*	–.33†	–.08
4. General Deviant Behavior in the Past Year	.41†	.54†	.36†		–.13	–.15*	.41†	.19*	.06		–.15	.29***
Conventional Behavior												
5. Church Attendance Frequency in the Past Year	.03	–.04	–.16	–.19*		.02	–.17	–.26**	–.33***	–.12		–.05
6. School Performance in the Past Year	–.28***	–.27***	–.37†	–.28***	.15		.07	–.16	.03	–.02	.08	
Year 3												
Problem Behavior												
1. Times Drunk in the Past Year		.22***	.34†	.31†	–.10	–.36†		.10	.18*	.19*	–.13	.01
2. Frequency of Marijuana Use in the Past 6 Months	.67†		.23***	.38†	–.08	–.14*	.36†		.34†	.34†	–.20**	.00
3. Frequency of Sexual Experience	.38†	.30***		.29†	–.05	–.08	.04	.20*		.20**	–.30***	–.19*
4. General Deviant Behavior in the Past Year	.41†	.34†	.37†		–.03	–.30†	.31***	.22**	.32***		–.10	–.10
Conventional Behavior												
5. Church Attendance Frequency in the Past Year	–.16*	–.11	–.19*	–.07		.20**	–.12	–.16	–.44†	–.20*		.01
6. School Performance in the Past Year	–.04	–.02	–.13	–.06	.15		.11	–.12	–.02	.06	.14	

[a]Correlations based on data from 102 men and 141 women
[b]Correlations based on data from 84 men and 100 women
*$p \leq .10$. ** $p \leq .05$. *** $p \leq .01$. †$p \leq .001$, two-tailed

Table 6.2 Maximum likelihood test for one common factor underlying problem behaviors by sex and sample in years 4 and 3

	High school				College			
	Men ($n=102$)		Women ($n=141$)		Men ($n=84$)		Women ($n=100$)	
Measure	Loading	h^2	Loading	h^2	Loading	h^2	Loading	h^2
Year 4								
Times Drunk in the Past Year	.46	.21	.31	.10	.73	.54	.28	.08
Frequency of Marijuana Use in the Past 6 Months	.60	.36	.33	.11	.35	.12	.46	.21
Frequency of Sexual Experience	.41	.17	.52	.27	.03	.00	.74	.55
General Deviant Behavior in the Past Year	.89	.80	.80	.63	.56	.31	.25	.06
Variance Portion	1.54		1.11		0.97		0.91	
% of Variance	38.6		27.8		24.2		22.7	
X^2 (2)	0.7 ($p=.72$)		2.0 ($p=.37$)		1.3 ($p=.51$)		1.6 ($p=.45$)	
Year 3								
Times Drunk in the Past Year	.88	.77	.52	.27	.54	.30	.25	.06
Frequency of Marijuana Use in the Past 6 Months	.75	.56	.51	.26	.53	.28	.66	.43
Frequency of Sexual Experience	.44	.20	.50	.25	.34	.12	.49	.24
General Deviant Behavior in the Past Year	.48	.23	.64	.40	.55	.31	.50	.25
Variance Portion	1.77		1.19		1.00		0.98	
% of Variance	44.1		29.8		25.0		24.6	
X^2 (2)	4.1 ($p=.13$)		3.1 ($p=.21$)		6.2 ($p=.05$)		2.2 ($p=.33$)	

Sexual Experience in the college male sample—were statistically significant by the Burt-Banks formula (Burt & Banks, 1947). These results were generally replicated in the analyses of the Year 3 data. In three of the four analyses in the replication year (Year 3), a single common factor accounted for the correlations among the problem behaviors. Only for the college sample men did the chi-square test indicate that the one-factor model failed to account for the observed correlations among the behaviors. The discrepancy was just large enough to reach significance.

Several other outcomes of these factor analyses should also be noted. First, the average percentage of the variance on the observed variables that was explained by the single common factor was considerably larger for the men than for the women in the high school analyses, and only slightly larger for the men than for the women in the analyses of the college data. Second, for both sexes and in both waves of data, this percentage was higher in the high school sample than in the comparable college sample. Third, there was considerable variation between the Year 4 and the Year 3 results in the size, if not in the significance, of the factor loadings for the different problem behaviors.

These analyses of the two separate waves of Year 3 and Year 4 data suggest that problem drinking, illicit drug use, precocious sexual behavior, and delinquent-type behavior do indeed reflect a single underlying factor in these samples of senior high school adolescents and college-age youth.

Study II

The second aim of the present investigation was to determine the generality of the factor-analytic results obtained in the high school sample in Study I for a more representative sample of adolescents, those who participated in the 1978 National Study of Adolescent Drinking. These data were collected by the Research Triangle Institute under the primary sponsorship of the National Institute on Alcohol Abuse and Alcoholism (Rachal et al., 1980).

Method

Overall design of the 1978 National Study of Adolescent Drinking. A sample of 5638 students in Grades 10 through 12 in the 48 contiguous states and the District of Columbia was drawn using a multistage stratified random sampling design. In each of 50 counties selected from strata that differed in geographic region and population size a sampling frame was established that consisted of all senior high schools, and at least one senior high school was selected in each county. A total of 74 different schools participated in the study. One classroom of 10th-, 11th-, and 12th- grade students was selected in each school, and all students in the selected classrooms were contacted and asked to participate in the survey. Self-administered questionnaires were completed in a classroom situation by 4918 students between March and April 1978. The overall response rate for the 1978 National Study of Adolescent Drinking was 86 % (see Rachal et al., 1980).

The resulting sample obtained for the 1978 national drinking study was 46 % male, and its self-reported ethnic distribution was white (Anglo), 72 %; black, 10 %; Spanish American, 5 %; Native American, 3 %; Asian American, 1 %; and other (or no answer), 9 %.

To increase the comparability between this sample and the high school sample examined in Study I, only data from the 11th- and 12th-grade students in the national sample were used in Study II. These were the same two grades that were involved in the Year 4 analyses of the local high school sample in Study I. There were 1208 boys and 1444 girls in these grades in the 1978 national sample data who also had scores on all of the behavior measures.[7]

Behavior measures. The 37-page questionnaire administered to the national sample contained abridged versions of the psychosocial and behavior measures of Problem Behavior Theory used in the earlier longitudinal study (Jessor & Jessor, 1977). The following behavior measures were included in this replication on a national sample of the factor analyses described in Study I: Number of Cigarettes Smoked per Day in the Last Month (range, 0–8 from *none* to *almost 3 packs a day*); Times Drunk in the Past Year (range, 0–8 from *none* to *weekly or more often*); Frequency of Marijuana Use in the Past Six Months (range, 1–10 from *never or not in past six months* to *every day*); Number of Other Illicit Drugs Ever Used (range, 0–7); General Deviant Behavior in the Past Year, a 12-item version of the longer scale used in the longitudinal study (range, 0–48; α=.80); Church Attendance Frequency in the Past Year (range, 1–7 from *have not gone* to *twice or more weekly*); and School Performance (range, 1–7; usual grades from *mostly Ds and Fs* to *mostly As*). Questions regarding sexual behavior could not be included in the national study questionnaire. All of these measures except the measure of smoking are described elsewhere (Jessor, Donovan, & Widmer, 1980).

Results

The correlations among the problem behavior measures and conventional behavior measures are presented in Table 6.3 for each sex separately. As may be seen, all of the correlations among the problem behaviors, between the problem behavior measures and the conventional behavior measures, and between the conventional behavior measures were statistically significant for both sexes.

Maximum likelihood tests for one common factor. Because models tested on large samples are often disconfirmed on the basis of essentially trivial perturbations in the data, the single-factor model was not tested using the full sample available for each sex. Instead, four small random samples of adolescents of each sex were selected

[7]The 4918 students in the national sample divided equally into 10th, 11th, and 12th graders. Of the 3279 students in the two older grade cohorts, 1540 were men and 1739 were women. When students who were missing scores on any of the behavior measures to be examined in the factor analyses were deleted from the sample, there were 1208 men (78 % of those in Grades 11 and 12) and 1444 women (83 % of those in Grades 11 and 12) remaining with complete data on the seven behavior measures.

Table 6.3 Correlations among selected measures of problem and conventional behavior by sex in 1978 National Sample Data (11th–12th graders only)

Measure	1	2	3	4	5	6	7
Problem Behavior							
1. Number of Cigarettes Smoked Per Day in the Last Month	–	.39	.42	.36	.40	–.24	–.24
2. Times Drunk in the Past Year	.32	–	.65	.53	.52	–.25	–.23
3. Frequency of Marijuana Use in the Past 6 Months	.34	.59	–	.58	.49	–.27	–.28
4. Number of Other Illicit Drugs Ever Used	.33	.43	.59	–	.43	–.26	–.21
5. General Deviant Behavior in the Past Year	.32	.46	.43	.36	–	–.20	–.28
Conventional Behavior							
6. Church Attendance Frequency in the Past Year	–.16	–.24	–.26	–.21	–.16	–	.17
7. School Performance	–.22	–.25	–.22	–.14	–.28	.12	–

Note: All correlations are statistically significant at the .001 level (two-tailed test). The lower triangular matrix contains the correlations for the men ($n=1208$) with no missing data; the upper triangular matrix contains the correlations for the women ($n=1444$).

from the larger sample. Ten-percent subsamples were used to obtain groups of approximately the same size as the sex groups studied in the local sample in Study I. The fit of the single-factor model was then tested in each of the eight random subsamples. Bartlett's test of sphericity showed that all of these matrices were appropriate for factor analysis.

The results of the eight maximum likelihood factor analyses are presented in Table 6.4. As may be seen, in all four analyses for each sex, the chi-square tests indicated that the singlefactor model can account for the correlations among this array of diverse problem behaviors. There were nonsignificant differences in each subsample between the observed correlations and the correlations predicted by the one-factor model. Of the 40 loadings of the problem behaviors on the underlying common factor, only one factor loading was below .3, and all were significant by the Burt-Banks formula. These results offer strong confirmation of the findings obtained from the local high school sample of adolescents in Study I.

Study III

The concern of the third study was the developmental generality of the previous findings from Studies I and II. Basically, the question was whether a similar syndrome of problem behavior would be evident in a sample of young adults in their middle to late 20s. The young adults, it will be remembered, were the same people who earlier had provided the data for the analyses presented in Study I.

Method

Behavior measures. In general, the measures assessed in young adulthood were similar to the measures assessed in the earlier phase of the longitudinal study. However, in recognition of the more mature, adult status of the participants by 1979 and 1981, some changes were made in the set of behavior measures examined: Two of the behavior measures used in Study I, School Performance and Frequency of Sexual Experience, were omitted, and a measure of the number of illicit drugs other than marijuana used in the past 6 months was substituted (drugs included stimulants, barbiturates, tranquilizers, psychedelic drugs, cocaine, heroin, other narcotic drugs). Measures included in the analyses of the young adult data were the following: Times Drunk in the Past Six Months (range, 0–90); Frequency of Marijuana Use in the Past Month (range, 0–60); Number of Other Illicit Drugs Used in the Past Six Months (range, 0–7); General Deviant Behavior in the Past Year, assessed by a shorter, 12-item index consisting of behaviors more appropriate to young adulthood (range, 0–12); and Church Attendance Frequency in the Past Year (range, 0–90). (Both the Times Drunk and Church Attendance measures were assessed in 1981 using categorical response options.)

As in Study I, separate analyses were carried out on each of the four Sex by Sample groups. In these young adult data, factor analyses based on the 1979 data were used as a check on the results of analyses of the 1981 data.

Table 6.4 Maximum likelihood tests for one common factor underlying problem behavior in four random 10 % subsamples selected from the 1978 National Study of Adolescent Drinking

	High school men								High school women							
	$n=105$		$n=113$		$n=136$		$n=129$		$n=145$		$n=148$		$n=156$		$n=141$	
Behavior Measure	Loading	h^2	Loading	h^2	Loading	h^2	Loading	h^2	Loading	h^2	Loading	h^2	Loading	h^2	Loading	h^2
Number of Cigarettes Smoked Per Day in the Last Month	.24	.06	.40	.16	.53	.28	.39	.15	.45	.20	.64	.41	.44	.19	.65	.43
Times Drunk in the Past Year	.62	.39	.65	.42	.74	.55	.61	.37	.90	.81	.73	.53	.78	.61	.77	.59
Frequency of Marijuana Use in the Past 6 Months	.85	.72	.90	.81	.82	.67	.78	.60	.80	.64	.86	.74	.74	.55	.82	.67
Number of Other Illicit Drugs Ever Used	.72	.53	.73	.53	.74	.55	.61	.37	.45	.20	.69	.47	.61	.37	.65	.42
General Deviant Behavior in the Past Year	.50	.25	.49	.24	.61	.38	.41	.17	.58	.33	.47	.23	.58	.33	.70	.49
Variance Portion	1.93		2.17		2.42		1.68		2.18		2.37		2.06		2.59	
% of Variance	38.7		43.4		48.4		33.5		43.7		47.4		41.3		51.9	
X^2 (5)	8.0 ($p=.16$)		8.2 ($p=.15$)		5.1 ($p=.40$)		5.5 ($p=.36$)		7.8 ($p=.17$)		5.0 ($p=.41$)		4.4 ($p=.49$)		5.1 ($p=.40$)	

Results

The Pearson correlations among the behaviors selected for inclusion in the young adult factor analyses are presented in Table 6.5 by sex and by sample for the 1981 data and for the 1979 data. For the high school sample data in both 1981 and 1979, the great majority of the correlations were statistically significant ($p < .05$). Of the four nonsignificant correlations, two reflected at least trends ($p < .10$) of a relation between Marijuana Use and Deviant Behavior for the women in both years. The measure of conventional behavior, Church Attendance Frequency, correlated in the negative direction, as expected, with all of the young adult problem behaviors, and most consistently with lower scores on the illicit drug use measures. For the college sample data, the correlations among the problem behaviors were strongest for the men in the 1981 data and weakest for this same group in the 1979 data. Only for the college sample men in 1981 did Times Drunk and Deviant Behavior correlate significantly with Frequency of Marijuana Use, and General Deviant Behavior failed to relate to the other problem behaviors in the 1979 data for the men. Although Church Attendance Frequency was negatively correlated with all but one of the problem behaviors, the relations generally were not statistically significant The eight young adult correlation matrices in Table 6.5 appeared appropriate for factor analysis. Bartlett's test of sphericity was highly significant ($p < .001$) in all cases.

Maximum likelihood tests for one common factor. The results of the maximum likelihood factor analyses of Times Drunk, Frequency of Marijuana Use, Number of Other Illicit Drugs Used, and Deviant Behavior are shown in Table 6.6. In both the key year (1981) and the replication year (1979), the chi-square tests of the discrepancy between the observed correlation matrix and the matrix predicted by the one-factor model were nonsignificant, supporting the hypothesis that one common factor subtends the correlations among the different behaviors.

All of the problem behavior measures loaded positively on the underlying common factor, and all of the loadings were significant except for two loadings in the 1979 data. In contrast to Study I, greater consonance occurred in Study III across data waves and subsamples in the relative magnitude of the factor loadings for the different problem behaviors. For example, Number of Other Illicit Drugs Used was found to be the behavior most strongly determined by the common factor in seven of the eight analyses, and Frequency of Marijuana Use was the next most strongly determined behavior in seven of the eight young adult analyses.

Discussion

The major aim of the present research was to test the hypothesis that the interrelations among different adolescent problem behaviors can be accounted for by a single common factor. This hypothesis was supported by a variety of maximum likelihood factor analyses carried out in three studies.

Table 6.5 Correlations among selected measures of Problem and Conventional Behavior in 1981 and 1979 by sex and sample

	High school sample men\women[a]					College sample men\women[b]				
Measure	1	2	3	4	5	1	2	3	4	5
1981										
Problem Behavior										
1. Times Drunk in the Past 6 Months		.20**	.38†	.22***	−.26***		.16	.43†	.54†	−.15
2. Frequency of Marijuana Use in the Past Month	.53†		.51†	.15*	−.17**	.35***		.24**	.07	−.08
3. Number of Other Illicit Drugs Used in the Past 6 Months	.52†	.55†		.29†	−.25***	.39†	.55†		.29***	−.15
4. General Deviant Behavior in the Past Year	.31***	28***	.46†		−.14*	.15	.37†	.33***		−.10
Conventional Behavior										
5. Church Attendance Frequency in the Past Year	−.33†	−.14	−.32***	−.13		−.17	−.07	−.30***	−.06	
1979										
Problem Behavior										
1. Times Drunk in the Past 6 Months		.05	.05	.22***	−.03		.16	.15	.29***	−.13
2. Frequency of Marijuana Use in the Past Month	.36†		.45†	.14*	−.17**	.10		.38†	.15	−.16
3. Number of Other Illicit Drugs Used in the Past 6 Months	.26***	.48†		.21***	−.22***	.37†	.38†		.21**	−.15
4. General Deviant Behavior in the Past Year	.26***	.24**	.37†		.26***	.07	.07	.07		−.23**
Conventional Behavior										
5. Church Attendance Frequency in the Past Year	−.11	−.25**	−.25**	−.08		−.12	−.20*	−.26**	.19*	

[a]Correlations based on data from 102 men and 141 women
[b]Correlations based on data from 84 men and 100 women
*$p \leq .10$. **$p \leq .05$. ***$p \leq .01$. †$p \leq .001$, two-tailed

Table 6.6 Maximum likelihood test of one common factor underlying behaviors by sex and sample in 1981 and 1979

	High school				College			
	Men (n=102)		Women (n=141)		Men (n=84)		Women (n=100)	
Measure	Loading	h^2	Loading	h^2	Loading	h^2	Loading	h^2
1981								
Times Drunk in the Past 6 Months	.68	.47	.41	.17	.47	.23	.88	.77
Frequency of Marijuana Use in the Past Month	.70	.49	.54	.30	.74	.55	.20	.04
Number of Other Illicit Drugs Used in the Past 6 Months	.79	.63	.92	.85	.75	.57	.50	.25
General Deviant Behavior in the Past Year	.50	.25	.32	.10	.45	.20	.61	.37
Variance Portion	1.84		1.42		1.55		1.42	
% of Variance	46.0		35.6		38.7		35.6	
X^2 (2)	4.2 (p=.12)		1.6 (p=.46)		1.0 (p=.60)		3.3 (p=.19)	
1979								
Times Drunk in the Past 6 Months	.46	.21	.10	.01	.37	.14	.33	.11
Frequency of Marijuana Use in the Past Month	.67	.45	.58	.33	.38	.14	.56	.32
Number of Other Illicit Drugs Used in the Past 6 Months	.70	.49	.77	.59	.99	.99	.61	.37
General Deviant Behavior in the Past Year	.47	.22	.28	.08	.07	.00	.37	.14
Variance Portion	1.37		1.01		1.28		0.93	
% of Variance	34.3		25.4		32.1		23.3	
X^2 (2)	3.8 (p=.15)		5.9 (p=.053)		0.5 (p=.78)		4.6 (p=.10)	

In Study I, the correlations among alcohol misuse, the use of marijuana, the commission of different delinquent-type behaviors, and precocious involvement in sexual intercourse were accounted for by a single underlying common factor. The observed correlations among these self-reported behaviors were not significantly different from the correlations predicted by the single-factor model. This result was found to demonstrate considerable generality across sex, across samples differing in educational level (high school vs. college), and across two different waves of longitudinal data within each subsample.

In Study II, factor analyses of data from a national sample of adolescents showed that the single-factor model is not limited only to Anglo middle-class adolescents but has generality for adolescents of widely differing socioeconomic and ethnic backgrounds from all over the country. These results, because they are based on data collected in 1978, also suggest that the single-factor explanation of the correlations among the different problem behaviors is not the result of a cohort effect, that is, it is not an artifact of the late-60s/early-70s "counter-culture."

In Study III, the results demonstrated the developmental generality of the earlier findings. A single common factor accounted for the correlations among several problem behaviors in the samples of young adults in their middle to late 20s who had participated previously in the Jessors' (1977) study of high school and college youth.

One interpretation of the present results is that they provide further support for the notion of a syndrome of problem behavior in both adolescence and young adulthood. Such support derives from the definition of a syndrome as "a set of behaviors believed to have a common cause or basis" (English & English, 1958) and from the capability of factor analysis to reveal the presence of underlying common causative factors.

Because factor analysis is based on correlational data, it cannot do more than suggest the nature of the underlying causal factor that accounts for the interrelations among the target behaviors. On the basis of our previous research, however, we can hypothesize that the common factor underlying the syndrome of problem behavior reflects a general dimension of *unconventionality*—in both personality and the social environment. Support for this interpretation of the underlying factor derives from several sources. First, previous analyses have shown that a consistent set of personality and social environment variables reflecting unconventionality correlates similarly with diverse adolescent behaviors such as marijuana use, problem drinking, delinquent-type behavior, and precocious sexual intercourse (Jessor & Jessor, 1977).[8] Similar findings have emerged from analyses of the data from both the 1974 and the 1978 National Study of Adolescent Drinking (Jessor, Chase, & Donovan, 1980;

[8] Involvement in each of these problem behaviors has been shown to be associated with the following psychosocial attributes: lower value on academic achievement; higher value on independence; greater value on independence relative to achievement; lower expectation for academic recognition; lower religiosity; greater tolerance of socially disapproved behavior; greater weight placed on the positive relative to the negative reasons for drinking, drug use, and sex; greater orientation toward friends than toward parents; less perceived compatibility of interests and values between parents and friends; greater perceived parental approval of problem behavior; and greater friends' approval and models for involvement in problem behavior.

Jessor, Donovan, & Widmer, 1980). Second, factor analyses found that a composite index of personality and social conventionality—indicated by greater religiosity, greater intolerance of deviance, more conservative sociopolitical attitudes, stricter friends' controls, fewer models and less approval for drug use, and more friend models for involvement with religion—loaded strongly on the underlying common factor in the opposite direction from that of the problem behavior measures in 12 of 12 analyses, and the common factor accounted for the intercorrelations among these variables in 10 of 12 analyses. (Analyses based on this composite measure were carried out on the Year 4 data from Study I and on the 1979 and 1981 young adult data from Study III.) Third, the conforming behavior measures of Church Attendance and School Performance were found to load in the negative direction on the common factor underlying the problem behaviors.[9]

Several important limitations of the present research must be mentioned. The first limitation derives from our exclusive reliance on self-report measures of behavior as the basic data for the analyses. Previous research that has compared self-reports of adolescent problem behaviors with official police records, reports of peer informants, and results of polygraph examinations generally supports the validity of such self-report behavior measures (Blackmore, 1974; Clark & Tifft, 1966; Gibson, Morrison, & West, 1970; Gold, 1966; Midanik, 1982). It is possible, however, that the use of these behavioral self-reports may have increased the likelihood of finding a single factor due to the influence of common method (common source) variance.

A second limitation of the present research lies in the nonrepresentative nature of the samples examined in Study I and Study III. Although this does constrain the generalizability of the findings beyond these samples, it does not limit the testing of theoretical or developmental issues.

The evidence in the young adult data that there is a syndrome of problem behavior implies a considerable degree of continuity between adolescence and young adulthood in the interrelations among the different problem behaviors. This continuity over time in the relations among the problem behaviors contrasts sharply with the evidence for noncontinuity in levels of involvement in these behaviors. For instance, Donovan, Jessor, and Jessor (1983) found that the majority of problem drinkers in these adolescent samples were no longer involved in abusive drinking as young adults. Together, these two different trends suggest that young adults may tend to disengage from involvement in multiple problem behaviors at the same time, rather than giving up their involvements one at a time as they grow older.

---

[9] In Study I, these loadings were statistically significant only for Church Attendance Frequency in the college sample analyses. In seven of the eight analyses, the chi-square tests indicated that the correlations among the problem behaviors and conforming behaviors could be accounted for by a single factor. In Study II, factor analyses in eight new random subsamples found that the conforming behaviors loaded negatively on the common factor in all cases. The chi-square tests, however, indicated a lack of fit with the single-factor model in three of the four male subsamples and in one of the female subsamples, which suggests that the conforming behaviors may constitute a correlated second factor for the men. In Study III, Church Attendance Frequency loaded negatively on the common factor in all eight analyses, and the chi-square tests showed that the single-factor model accounted for the data in all cases.

Further research aimed at understanding the structure of behavior among adolescents is clearly needed. For example, while adolescent alcohol misuse, drug abuse, cigarette smoking, and precocious sexual intercourse are all problem behaviors, they are also behaviors with important implications for adolescent health and well-being (Califano, 1979). Little is currently known, however, regarding their relations to the wider array of health-related behaviors among adolescents, for example, eating and exercise behavior. It would be important for future research to determine the perimeter of a possibly larger syndrome of health-related behavior in adolescence.

The factor analyses presented in this article imply that a sizable proportion of the common variance among the different problem behaviors can be accounted for by their common relations to unconventionality in personality and social attributes. But the behaviors may be correlated for other reasons as well, for example, because they are seen by young people as substitutable or interchangeable means of achieving valued goals; because they are learned together and continue to be performed together; or because of linkages in the social ecology of adolescence (in certain socially structured situations there is considerable peer approval, pressure, and expectation for involvement in multiple problem behaviors such as alcohol use, cigarette smoking, marijuana use, and precocious sex in a single setting, such as an unchaperoned party). Research examining these alternative explanations of the structure of problem behavior could provide a more finely textured understanding of adolescent behavior.

Finally, the implication of the findings in this article for prevention programs should be emphasized. Prevention programs may well benefit by broadening their focus beyond their traditional concern with individual problem behaviors, for example, drug use, drunk driving, or unprotected sexual activity. Given the interrelations that obtain among drug abuse, problem drinking, cigarette smoking, and delinquent behavior, such programs might well focus more generally on the larger behavior syndrome.

Acknowledgments This research was carried out as part of a larger project, the Young Adult Follow-Up Study (R. Jessor, principal investigator), which was funded by National Institute on Alcohol Abuse and Alcoholism Grant A A03745. The research was carried out under the aegis of the Research Program on Problem Behavior in the Institute of Behavioral Science of the University of Colorado at Boulder.

We would like to acknowledge the contributions of Frances Costa and Lee Jessor to the planning and collection of the young adult data used in this study. We thank J. Valley Rachal, who directed the 1978 National Study of Adolescent Drinking, for providing us with a copy of the raw data. We are grateful to Frances Costa, John Finney, and Ron Hays for their suggestions on an earlier draft of this article.

References

Bachman, J. G., O'Malley, P. M., & Johnston, L. D. (1980). *Correlates of drug use, part I: Selected measures of background, recent experiences, and lifestyle orientations* (Monitoring the Future Occasional Paper 8). Ann Arbor, MI: Institute for Social Research.

Bachman, J. G., O'Malley, P. M., & Johnston, L. D. (1984). Drug use among young adults: The impacts of role status and social environment. *Journal of Personality and Social Psychology, 47*, 629–645.

Bartlett, M. S. (1950). Tests of significance in factor analysis. *British Journal of Psychology, 3*, 77–85.
Blackmore, J. (1974). The relationship between self-reported delinquency and official convictions amongst adolescent boys. *British Journal of Criminology, 14*, 172–176.
Block, J. R., & Goodman, N. (1978). Illicit drug use and consumption of alcohol, tobacco, and over-the-counter medicine among adolescents. *International Journal of the Addictions, 13*, 933–946.
Burt, C., & Banks, C. (1947). A factor analysis of body measurements for British adult males. *Annals of Eugenics, 13*, 238–256.
Califano, J. A., Jr. (1979). *Healthy people: The Surgeon General's report on health promotion and disease prevention*. Washington, DC: U.S. Department of Health, Education, and Welfare.
Clark, J. P., & Tifft, L. L. (1966). Polygraph and interview validation of self-reported deviant behavior. *American Sociological Review, 31*, 516–523.
Donovan, J. E., & Jessor, R. (1978). Adolescent problem drinking: Psychosocial correlates in a national sample study. *Journal of Studies on Alcohol, 39*, 1506–1524.
Donovan, J. E., Jessor, R., & Jessor, L. (1983). Problem drinking in adolescence and young adulthood: A follow-up study. *Journal of Studies on Alcohol, 44*, 109–137.
English, H. B., & English, A. C. (1958). *A comprehensive dictionary of psychological and psychoanalytical terms*. New York: David McKay.
Gibson, H. B., Morrison, S., & West, D. J. (1970). The confession of known offenses in response to a self-reported delinquency schedule. *British Journal of Criminology, 10*, 277–280.
Gold, M. (1966). Undetected delinquent behavior. *Journal of Research in Crime and Delinquency, 3*, 21–46.
Gove, W. R., Geerken, M., & Hughes, M. (1979). Drug use and mental health among a representative sample of young adults. *Social Forces, 58*, 572–590.
Hays, R. D., Widaman, K. F., DiMatteo, M. R., & Stacy, A. W. (1987). Structural- equation models of current drug use: Are appropriate models so simple(x)? *Journal of Personality and Social Psychology, 52*(1), 134–144.
Hindelang, M. J. (1971). Age, sex, and the versatility of delinquent involvements. *Social Problems, 18*, 522–535.
Hitachi, T. (1969). *Causes of delinquency*. Berkeley: University of California Press.
Huba, G. J. (1983). Cross-validation of a drug use causal model in the Columbia longitudinal study data. *Bulletin of the Society of Psychologists in Addictive Behaviors, 2*, 128–132.
Huba, G. J., & Bentler, P. M. (1979). Phencyclidine use in high school: Tests of models. *Journal of Drug Education, 9*, 285–291.
Huba, G. J., & Bentler, P. M. (1982). On the usefulness of latent variable causal modeling in testing theories of naturally occurring events (including adolescent drug use): A rejoinder to Martin. *Journal of Personality and Social Psychology, 43*, 604–611.
Huba, G. J., Wingard, J. A., & Bentler, P. M. (1981). A comparison of two latent variable causal models for adolescent drug use. *Journal of Personality and Social Psychology, 40*, 180–193.
Hundleby, J. D. (1979). *Individual and environmental predictors and correlates of adolescent drug-related behaviour* (Modified version of final report to the Non-medical Use of Drugs Directorate, Health and Welfare, Canada). Guelph, Ontario: University of Guelph.
Istvan, J., & Matarazzo, J. D. (1984). Tobacco, alcohol, and caffeine use: A review of their interrelationships. *Psychological Bulletin, 95*, 301–326.
Jessor, R. (1983). The stability of change: Psychosocial development from adolescence to young adulthood. In D. Magnusson & V. Allen (Eds.), *Human development: An interactional perspective* (pp. 321–341). New York: Academic Press.
Jessor, R., Chase, J. A., & Donovan, J. E. (1980). Psychosocial correlates of marijuana use and problem drinking in a national sample of adolescents. *American Journal of Public Health, 70*, 604–613.
Jessor, R., Costa, F., Jessor, L., & Donovan, J. E. (1983). Time of first intercourse: A prospective study. *Journal of Personality and Social Psychology, 44*, 608–626.

Jessor, R., Donovan, J. E., & Widmer, K. (1980). *Psychosocial factors in adolescent alcohol and drug use: The 1978 National Sample Study and the 1974–78 Panel Study*. Boulder: Institute of Behavioral Science, University of Colorado.

Jessor, R., & Jessor, S. L. (1977). *Problem behavior and psychosocial development: A longitudinal study of youth*. New York: Academic Press.

Jessor, R., & Jessor, S. L. (1984). Adolescence to young adulthood: A twelve-year prospective study of problem behavior and psychosocial development. In S. A. Mednick, M. Harway, & K. M. Finello (Eds.), *Handbook of longitudinal research in the United States* (Vol. 2, pp. 34–61). New York: Praeger.

Johnson, B. D. (1973). *Marihuana users and drug subcultures*. New York: Wiley.

Johnston, L. D. (1973). *Drugs and American youth: A report from the Youth in Transition Project*. Ann Arbor, MI: Institute for Social Research.

Kandel, D. B. (1984). Marijuana users in young adulthood. *Archives of General Psychiatry, 41*, 200–209.

Mechanic, D., & Cleary, P. D. (1980). Factors associated with the maintenance of positive health behavior. *Preventive Medicine, 9*, 805–814.

Midanik, L. (1982). The validity of self-reported alcohol consumption and alcohol problems: A literature review. *British Journal of Addiction, 77*, 357–382.

Miller, J. D., Cisin, I. H., Gardner-Keaton, H., Harrell, A. V., Wirtz, P. W., Abelson, H. I., et al. (1983). *National survey on drug abuse: Main findings 1982 (DHHS Publication No. ADM 83-1263)*. Rockville, MD: National Institute on Drug Abuse.

Nie, N. H., Hull, C. H., Jenkins, J. G., Steinbrenner, K., & Bent, D. H. (1975). *SPSS: Statistical package for the social sciences* (2nd ed.). New York: McGraw-Hill.

O'Donnell, J. A., Voss, H. L., Clayton, R. R., Statin, G. T., & Room, R. (1976). *Young men and drugs. A nationwide survey* (DHEW Publication No. ADM 76311). Washington, DC: U.S. Government Printing Office.

Prendergast, T. J., Jr., & Schaefer, E. S. (1974). Correlates of drinking and drunkenness among high school students. *Quarterly Journal of Studies on Alcohol, 35*, 232–242.

Rachal, J. V., Guess, L. L., Hubbard, R. L., Maisto, S. A., Cavanaugh, E. R., Waddell, R., et al. (1980). *Adolescent drinking behavior, volume I: The extent and nature of adolescent alcohol and drug use: The 1974 and 1978 National Sample Studies*. Research Triangle Park, NC: Research Triangle Institute.

Single, E., Kandel, D., & Faust, R. (1974). Patterns of multiple drug use in high school. *Journal of Health and Social Behavior, 15*, 344–357.

Wechsler, H. (1976). Alcohol intoxication and drug use among teenagers. *Journal of Studies on Alcohol, 37*, 1672–1677.

Wechsler, H., & Thum, D. (1973). Teen-age drinking, drug use, and social correlates. *Quarterly Journal of Studies on Alcohol, 34*, 1220–1227.

Weitman, M., Scheble, R. O., Johnson, K. G., & Abbey, H. (1972). Survey of adolescent drug use: 3. *Correlations among use of drugs. American Journal of Public Health, 62*, 166–170.

Zucker, R. A., & Barron, F. H. (1973). Parental behaviors associated with problem drinking and antisocial behavior among adolescent males. In M. E. Chafetz (Ed.), *Proceedings of the First Annual Alcoholism Conference of the National Institute on Alcohol Abuse and Alcoholism* (DHEW Publication No. NIH 74-675, pp. 276–296). Washington, DC: U.S. Government Printing Office.

Zucker, R. A., & Devoe, C. I. (1975). Life history characteristics associated with problem drinking and antisocial behavior in adolescent girls: A comparison with male findings. In R. D. Wirt, G. Winokur, & M. Rolf (Eds.), *Life history research in psychopathology* (Vol. 4, pp. 109–134). Minneapolis: University of Minnesota Press.

Chapter 7
Replicating the Co-Variation of Adolescent Problem Behavior

John E. Donovan, Richard Jessor, and Frances M. Costa

A replication of an earlier study (Donovan & Jessor, 1985) of the structure of interrelations among a number of problem behaviors was carried out in a sample of adolescents from the general population. Previous research has shown substantial positive relations among a variety of adolescent problem behaviors, including alcohol use, cigarette smoking, marijuana use, use of other illicit drugs, delinquent behavior, and precocious sexual intercourse (e.g., Bachman, O'Malley, & Johnston, 1980; Hundleby, 1987; Jessor & Jessor, 1977; Zucker & Barron, 1973). Problem behaviors are socially defined by the norms of conventional society as undesirable for adolescents to engage in and involve the possibility of negative social sanctions.

In a longitudinal study of a sample of senior high school students and a sample of college students, Jessor and Jessor (1977) found that adolescent problem behaviors correlated positively with each other and correlated negatively with conventional behaviors, such as church attendance. The adolescent problem behaviors were also similar in their correlations with an array of personality and perceived social environment variables reflecting unconventionality in the social-psychological framework of Problem Behavior Theory. On the basis of these findings, Jessor and Jessor proposed that drinking, problem drinking, marijuana use, delinquent behavior, and precocious sexual intercourse may constitute a syndrome of problem behavior in adolescence.

Reprinted with permission from:
Donovan, J. E., Jessor, R., & Costa, F. M. (1988). Syndrome of problem behavior in adolescence: A replication. *Journal of Consulting and Clinical Psychology, 56*(5), 762–765.

J.E. Donovan
University of Pittsburgh, School of Medicine, Pittsburgh, USA

R. Jessor (✉)
Institute of Behavioral Science, University of Colorado at Boulder, Boulder, CO 80309, USA
e-mail: jessor@Colorado.edu

F.M. Costa
University of Colorado Boulder, Boulder, CO 80309, USA

R. Jessor, *The Origins and Development of Problem Behavior Theory*,
Advancing Responsible Adolescent Development,
DOI 10.1007/978-3-319-40886-6_7

Later analyses of these same data provided further support for the notion of such a syndrome. Maximum-likelihood factor analyses established that a single underlying common factor accounted for the intercorrelations among this set of problem behaviors in both the high school and the college study data, for both genders, in two independent waves of longitudinal data: 1971 and 1972 data for the high school sample, and 1972 and 1973 data for the college sample (Donovan & Jessor, 1985).

The present article assessed the degree of support for a syndrome of problem behavior among adolescents 13 years later, in 1985. Over this time interval, there has been a change in both the prevalence of and the normative beliefs about various problem behaviors (e.g., greater social acceptance of marijuana use, increased societal concern with alcohol abuse, especially drinking and driving, and more accepting attitudes about sex). Such changes may have influenced the structure of relations among the behaviors of adolescents.

Method

Study Design and Procedures

A stratified sampling frame was used to select a sample of male and female students in Grades 7–12 on the basis of school and grade attended from the 11 secondary schools in a single school district in northeastern Colorado. The district serves a number of urban and rural communities with a total population of around 72,000 residents and 7000 secondary school students.

Active parental consent was requested for students' participation in the research. Of the 3010 parents contacted by mail, 1667 (55 %) returned signed consent forms. This level of response is similar to that obtained in other studies in which active consent has been sought from parents (see Jessor & Jessor, 1977; Lueptow, Mueller, Hammes, & Master, 1977; Severson & Ary, 1983).

Data were collected between mid-November and mid-December of 1985. Anonymous questionnaires were filled out in large group settings (e.g., in the cafeteria). The questionnaires were distributed and collected by members of the research team. Each student was given a token payment of $5.

A total of 1588 students completed questionnaires, constituting 95 % of those who had received parental permission to participate and 53 % of those originally sampled. Of the 1588 participants, 83 % were White, 8 % were Hispanic, 5 % were Native American, 2 % were Asian American, and 0.4 % were Black. The majority of the students came from middle-class backgrounds, and most (70 %) lived in intact families. The analyses presented here are based on the self-reported behaviors of the 162 male and 226 female participants in Grades 11 and 12 (the grades assessed in 1972) who had scores on all of the behavior measures. These 11–12th-graders constituted 94 % and 92 %, respectively, of all participating male and female students in these grades.

Measures of Problem Behavior and Conventional Behavior

The 1985 Health Questionnaire was 29 pages long and was computer scanned and scored. Average time to complete the questionnaire was about 42 min for the senior high school participants. Many of the measures in the questionnaire had originally been developed to test the usefulness of Problem Behavior Theory (Jessor & Jessor, 1977) in accounting for variation in adolescent problem and conventional behaviors. The behavior measures used here are, for the most part, slightly modified versions of those original measures.

The four problem behaviors of problem drinking, marijuana use, delinquent-type behavior, and sexual intercourse were assessed by (a) times drunk in the past 6 months as gauged by the frequency of having been drunk or "very, very high" on alcohol (*never* to *more than twice a week*); (b) the frequency of marijuana use in the past 6 months (*never* to *every day*); (c) general deviant behavior as measured by a 10-item summative scale assessing how often in the past 6 months respondents had engaged in norm-violative activities, such as shoplifting, property destruction, fighting, and lying (score range = 0–60; Cronbach's alpha = .82); and (d) sexual intercourse experience, a dichotomous measure (coded 0 vs. 1) of virgin/nonvirgin status.

Two measures of conventional behavior were also included in the correlation analyses for purposes of discriminant validity; Church attendance frequency was assessed by a single question asking how often in the past year religious services had been attended (from *none* to *more than once a week*), and school performance was assessed by a single question concerning the grades earned in the preceding academic year (from *mostly D's and F's* to *mostly A's*).

In the maximum-likelihood factor analyses, the hypothesis was tested that a single common factor would account for the correlations among the problem behaviors. If this one-factor model is appropriate, the observed correlation between any two of the behaviors would be equal to the product of the estimated loadings of the behaviors on the common factor. The Jöreskog factor analysis procedure, available as part of the Statistical Package for the Social Sciences, Cyber Version 8.3 (Nie, Hull, Jenkins, Steinbrenner, & Bent, 1975), was used to compute large-sample chi-square tests of the discrepancy between the matrices of observed and predicted correlations among the problem behaviors. A nonsignificant ($p > .05$) chi-square value would provide evidence in support of the hypothesis of a single common factor and would replicate the results found in the earlier 1972 data; a significant chi-square value, on the other hand, would suggest that more than one common factor underlies the relations among the problem behaviors.

Results and Discussion

The Pearson correlations on which the factor analyses were based are presented in Table 7.1 for both the male and female participants separately. All four problem behavior measures correlated significantly and in the positive direction for both

Table 7.1 Correlations among measures of problem behavior and conventional behavior by gender

	High school male\female participants[a]					
Measure	1	2	3	4	5	6
Problem behavior						
1. Times drunk in past 6 months		.41*	.45*	.35*	−.28*	−.39*
2. Frequency of marijuana use in past 6 months	.57*		.38*	.33*	−.25*	−.25*
3. General deviant behavior in past 6 months	.53*	.46*		.22*	−.07	−.24*
4. Sexual intercourse experience	.50*	.35*	.35*		−.20*	−.36*
Conventional behavior						
5. Church attendance frequency in past year	−.09	−.31*	−.10	−.29*		.20*
6. School performance in previous academic year	−.28*	−.28*	−.30*	−.27*	.08	

Note. Due to the large number of correlations for each gender, an alpha of .0033 (two-tailed) was used to test the significance of each correlation. This alpha also satisfies the requirement of setting the Type I experimentwise error rate at .10. *Ns* = 162 for male participants, 226 for female participants
[a]Correlations for male participants are reported in the lower left triangular matrix; correlations for female participants are reported in the upper right triangular matrix
* $p < .002$ (two-tailed)

Table 7.2 Maximum-likelihood test for one common factor underlying the relations among four adolescent problem behaviors by gender

	Male participants ($n = 162$)		Female participants ($n = 226$)	
Measure	Loading	h^2	Loading	h^2
Times drunk in past 6 months	.85	.72	.74	.54
Frequency of marijuana use in past 6 months	.67	.45	.62	.38
General deviant behavior in past 6 months	.63	.40	.59	.35
Sexual intercourse experience	.57	.33	.48	.23
Variance portion	1.90		1.50	
% of variance	47.5		37.4	
$X^2(2)$	1.41 ($p = .495$)		2.54 ($p = .281$)	

genders. More frequent involvement in one of the problem behaviors was associated with more frequent involvement in the other problem behaviors.

The discriminant validity correlations between the four problem behaviors and the two conventional behaviors were all in the negative direction, as expected. School performance correlated negatively and significantly with each of the problem behaviors, whereas church attendance correlated negatively and significantly with marijuana use and sexual intercourse for both genders and with drunkenness for the male participants only.

Bartlett's test of sphericity was significant ($p < .0001$) for the problem behavior correlation matrices for both genders, indicating that these matrices are appropriate for use in factor analyses. The Kaiser-Meyer-Olkin measure of sampling adequacy was also satisfactory for both matrices: .76 for the male participants, .72 for the female participants (see Dziuban & Shirkey, 1974).

The results of the maximum-likelihood factor analyses are presented in Table 7.2. For neither the male nor the female participants were the chi-square values even close to significance. Thus, there were no statistically significant discrepancies between the observed correlation matrix and the matrix of correlations predicted by the one-factor model for either gender. It follows, then, that only a single common factor is needed to account for the correlations among the problem behaviors. All four of the problem behaviors had high, positive, statistically significant loadings on the underlying common factor for both genders. As may be seen, the loadings of the different problem behaviors on the underlying factor were proportional for the male and female participants, indicating the same relative determination of the behaviors by the common factor for both genders. The ordering of the behaviors, from most to least determined by the common factor, was times drunk, marijuana use, general deviance, and sexual experience. Somewhat more of the variation on the problem behavior measures was due to the common factor for the male (47.5 %) than for the female participants (37.4 %).

These results replicate our earlier findings. The replication is all the more compelling considering that 13 years have passed since the earlier study, that the measures used to assess the problem behaviors are different, and that the prevalence and social context of the adolescent problem behaviors have also changed.

This replication of the earlier factor-analytic results provides further evidence supporting the concept of a syndrome of problem behavior in adolescence. The nature of the underlying common factor that accounts for the existence of the syndrome is not revealed by these factor analyses, however. As in the earlier article, we hypothesize that the underlying common factor reflects a general dimension of conventionality/unconventionality in both personality and the social environment. Support for such an interpretation derives from the consistent correlations of the personality and social environment variables of Problem Behavior Theory with each of the problem behaviors as well as with a summary index of the number of problem behaviors involved in (alcohol use, problem drinking, cigarette smoking, marijuana use, use of other illicit drugs, delinquent-type behavior, and sexual intercourse). In the 1985 data, multiple correlations of .80 and .71 were obtained for the senior high school male and female participants, respectively, when using the variables of Problem Behavior Theory to account for variation on the summary problem behavior index.

A dichotomous measure of virgin/nonvirgin status was used in the present analyses to maintain consistency with the 1972 data. When an available measure of the frequency of sexual intercourse in the past year was used in the analyses instead, there was little difference in the results. A single common factor still accounted for the correlations among the various problem behaviors for both genders (chi-square values were again far from significant at $p = .775$ and $p = .232$ for the male and female participants, respectively).

Although the present findings replicate those of the earlier study, it is possible that the results were affected by two aspects of the research method. As in most survey research on adolescent problem behavior, those adolescents who took part were likely to have been more conventional than those who did not. This may have truncated the distributions on the problem behaviors, thereby attenuating the resulting correlations. At the same time, however, reliance on a common method of data collection, the use of self-reports of behavior, may have inflated the correlations among the problem behaviors. Given that these influences on the correlations among the behaviors are opposing, it is difficult to estimate the extent to which the obtained correlations may be biased.

The variance accounted for by the single, underlying factor (47 % of the total variance for the male participants, 37 % for the female participants) is larger than that accounted for in the 1972 data (39 % and 28 %, respectively). The variance on the problem behavior measures that was not determined by the common factor may be due to such influences as measurement error or unreliability and differences among the behaviors in their perceived psychological functions or meanings and in their degree of peer support.

This replication of the syndrome of problem behavior in adolescence suggests the need for further research to understand the structure of relations among other domains of behavior. For example, analyses of our data demonstrate that there are consistent relations between adolescent problem behaviors, on the one hand, and both health-enhancing and health-compromising behaviors, on the other. Little is known, however, about the structure of these behavioral relations or about the development of such structure. Additional knowledge in this area ought to have substantial implications for the design of prevention and intervention programs for adolescents.

References

Bachman, J. G., O'Malley, P. M., & Johnston, L. D. (1980). *Correlates of drug use: Part I. Selected measures of background, recent experiences, and lifestyle orientations* (Monitoring the Future Occasional Paper 8). Ann Arbor, MI: Institute for Social Research.

Donovan, J. E., & Jessor, R. (1985). Structure of problem behavior in adolescence and young adulthood. *Journal of Consulting and Clinical Psychology, 53*, 890–904.

Dziuban, C. D., & Shirkey, E. C. (1974). When is a correlation matrix appropriate for factor analysis? Some decision rules. *Psychological Bulletin, 81*, 358–361.

Hundleby, J. D. (1987). Adolescent drug use in a behavioral matrix: A confirmation and comparison of the sexes. *Addictive Behaviors, 12*, 103–112.

Jessor, R., & Jessor, S. L. (1977). *Problem behavior and psychosocial development: A longitudinal study of youth*. New York: Academic Press.

Lueptow, L., Mueller, S., Hammes, R., & Master, L. (1977). The impact of informed consent regulations on response rate and response set. *Sociological Methods and Research, 6*, 183–204.

Nie, N. H., Hull, C. H., Jenkins, J. G., Steinbrenner, K., & Bent, D. H. (1975). *SPSS: Statistical package for the social sciences* (2nd ed.). New York: McGraw-Hill.

Severson, H. H., & Ary, D. V. (1983). Sampling bias due to consent procedures with adolescents. *Addictive Behaviors, 8*, 433–437.

Zucker, R. A., & Barron, F. H. (1973). Parental behaviors associated with problem drinking and antisocial behavior among adolescent males. In M. E. Chafetz (Ed.), Proceedings of the First Annual Alcoholism Conference of the National Institute on Alcohol Abuse and Alcoholism (DHEW Publication No. NIH 74-675, pp. 276–296). Washington, DC: U.S. Government Printing Office.

Chapter 8
Problem Behavior Theory and Adolescent Risk Behavior: A Re-Formulation

Richard Jessor

There is a growing awareness that American society is squandering its most precious asset, its youth. Large segments of our young people are growing up in circumstances of such limited resources and pervasive adversity that, for many of them, their health, their development, indeed their lives as a whole, are certain to be severely—and perhaps irretrievably—compromised. Those who manage to supervene these conditions and "make it" in the larger society deserve an accolade for heroism. Those, on the other hand, whose lives have been deflected from a trajectory of possibility can only be seen as its victims. These remarks about the larger social context are a deliberate prolegomenon to my discussion of adolescents and risk; in too much of the discourse in this field there has been a failure to recognize the fundamental role of socially organized poverty, inequality, and discrimination in producing and maintaining a population of at-risk youth. This concern with the larger society will emerge later on from the logic of the conceptual analysis of risk.

The key task for this paper is to sketch out a conceptual framework that might facilitate both understanding of and action in the arena of adolescent risk. Pursuit of that objective will involve a brief exploration of recent developments in epidemiology, particularly the emergence of behavioral epidemiology, and in social/developmental psychology, particularly its application to adolescent problem behavior. There is an increasing consonance between these disparate fields.

Reprinted with permission from:
Jessor, R. (1991). Risk behavior in adolescence: A psychosocial framework for understanding and action. *Journal of Adolescent Health, 12*(8), 597–605.

R. Jessor (✉)
Institute of Behavioral Science, University of Colorado at Boulder, Boulder, CO, USA
e-mail: jessor@Colorado.edu

R. Jessor, *The Origins and Development of Problem Behavior Theory*,
Advancing Responsible Adolescent Development,
DOI 10.1007/978-3-319-40886-6_8

The exploration begins with some considerations about the basic notion of *risk* itself; it then turns to an examination of the organization of adolescent risk behavior and the utility of the concept of *life-style*. It leads next into a general conceptual framework for understanding risk behavior and an explication of its content. Finally, some implications of the conceptual framework for action, in terms of prevention/intervention, will be noted. I have chosen not to review the literature in the field but, instead, to distill a perspective from several decades of theoretical and empirical work on these issues. Where useful, illustrative data will be drawn from our own research.

A Psychosocial Concept of Risk

In the tradition of epidemiology, the use of the concept of risk has been essentially biomedical, reflecting a concern for adverse outcomes related to morbidity and mortality. The epidemiological search has been to locate agents or conditions that are associated with an increased probability of outcomes that compromise health, quality of life, or life itself. Such agents or conditions are referred to as *risk factors*, and the search for such factors has kept its focus primarily on biology and, to some extent, on the physical environment as well. Biological risk factors, such as high serum cholesterol level and hypertension, have been linked to increased probability of cardiovascular disease; cervical dysplasia to cancer; abnormalities in trisomy 21 to Down syndrome. Various physical environment risk factors such as radiation, lead, or contaminated water have also been linked to adverse health outcomes and to death. The identification of risk factors has been a major achievement of epidemiology; it not only constitutes an initial step in establishing causal understanding but often suggests a locus for effective intervention.

More recently, the epidemiological search for risk factors for disease and illness, especially for the chronic diseases, has expanded into two new domains, social environment and behavior. With respect to the social environment, considerable attention has been given, for example, to such risk factors as stress and its implications for heart disease. The availability of and access to alcohol and tobacco, yet another aspect of the social environment, have been implicated as risk factors for cirrhosis and lung cancer. But perhaps the most reverberating development in epidemiology has been the new awareness of *behavior* as a risk factor, and the accompanying elaboration of the subdiscipline of behavioral epidemiology. It is increasingly apparent that much of the burden of illness—heart disease and stroke, cancer, liver disease, unintended injury, human immunodeficiency virus (HIV) infection—can be linked to patterns of human behavior. Eating behavior, sedentary behavior, drinking behavior, driving after drinking, smoking behavior, unprotected sexual intercourse, unsanitary practices, and other such actions can, it is now clear, compromise health and safety.

Insofar as behaviors constitute risk factors for morbidity and mortality, the challenge for epidemiology is to move beyond its usual biomedical focus and address a new task, the understanding of behavior and its antecedents and consequences. It is in undertaking this enterprise that epidemiology has begun to find a confluence with social/developmental psychology. For the latter, of course, the understanding of social behavior has been a traditional and important raison d'être.

The incorporation of behaviors into the rubric of risk factors entails a reformulation of thinking about the very concept of risk and about what is at risk. First, it requires that the traditional restriction of the concept of risk to biomedical outcomes alone be loosened. Although behaviors do indeed have biomedical consequences, they also eventuate in social and personal or psychological outcomes. The behavior of, say, marijuana smoking by an adolescent may well increase the probability of pulmonary disease, but it also may increase the probability of legal sanctions or conflict with parents or loss of interest in school or sense of personal guilt and anxiety. These latter are psychosocial outcomes or consequences that are linked, simultaneously, to the very same risk behavior. A *psychosocial* understanding of risk, when behaviors are risk factors, requires attention to all of their potential outcomes or consequences, not just to those that are biomedical.

Second, the reformulation requires that the restriction of the concept of risk to adverse, negative, or undesirable outcomes be loosened. Returning to the preceding example, it is clear that some of the outcomes or consequences of the behavioral risk factor of marijuana smoking can be positive, desirable, and sought by adolescents. Smoking marijuana can lead, for example, to social acceptance by peers and to a subjective sense of autonomy and maturity. When behaviors are risk factors, the notion of risk needs to be expanded to encompass positive or desired outcomes as well as those that are adverse or negative. A psychosocial reformulation of risk calls for a thorough cost *and* benefit analysis of risk factors rather than the traditional preoccupation with their potential costs alone. Behavior, including risk behavior, is clearly influenced by both.

The bankruptcy of the exhortation "Just Say No!" is evident in the failure to acknowledge that drug use and other risk behaviors can serve important social and personal functions for adolescents and are unlikely to be abandoned in the absence of alternatives that can provide similar satisfactions. Considerable research has shown that adolescent risk behaviors are functional, purposive, instrumental, and goal-directed and that these goals are often central to normal adolescent development. Smoking, drinking, illicit drug use, risky driving, or early sexual activity can be instrumental in gaining peer acceptance and respect; in establishing autonomy from parents; in repudiating the norms and values of conventional authority; in coping with anxiety, frustration, and anticipation of failure; or in affirming maturity and marking a transition out of childhood and toward a more adult status. There is nothing perverse, irrational, or psychopathological about such goals. Rather, they are characteristic of ordinary psychosocial development, and their centrality helps to explain why risk behaviors that serve such functions are so intractable to change. In failing to allocate resources to promote alternative behaviors that can serve the same goals but are less health- and life-compromising for adolescents, the "Just Say No!" campaign revealed its moral cynicism.

The concept of psychosocial risk implicates, and is concerned with, the entire range of personal development and social adaptation in adolescence. Thus, *what* is at risk from engaging in risk behavior includes, but far transcends, physical health and physical growth. Risk behaviors can jeopardize the accomplishment of normal developmental tasks, the fulfillment of expected social roles, the acquisition of essential skills, the achievement of a sense of adequacy and competence, and the appropriate preparation for transition to the next stage in the life trajectory, young adulthood. The term *risk behavior* refers, then, to any behavior that can compromise these psychosocial aspects of successful adolescent development. Substance abuse, withdrawal from school involvement, unprotected sexual intercourse, driving after drinking, and engaging in violence are some obvious examples.

It should be noted that I have not been using the term *risk-taking behavior.* I am concerned that the latter has been responsible for a certain amount of terminological mischief in the field. Its wide currency is unfortunate because it eliminates the problematic nature of adolescent risk behavior and tends to foreclose further inquiry. When referred to as risk-taking behavior, risk behavior is already "explained." That is, it is accounted for simply by the taking of risks, the satisfaction or thrill of engaging in something risky. There is an associated unfortunate tendency as well, and that is to characterize adolescents as "risk-takers." This not only results in a bit of tautological thinking that further confounds explanation but it also divests the social context of any contributory role.

The concept of risk-taking behavior is certainly appropriate for that subset of risk behaviors that entail a conscious awareness of the risk or danger involved and a deliberate seeking for the thrill that issues from the uncertainty of beating the odds. Playing the game of "chicken" on the highway, taking chances on avoiding detection during certain delinquent acts, or pursuing activities like rock climbing may be examples. But the larger class of adolescent risk behavior simply does not lend itself to that kind of analysis. Few adolescents continue cigarette smoking for the thrill of seeing whether they can avoid pulmonary disease; few engage in unprotected sexual intercourse for the thrill of beating the odds of contracting a sexually transmitted disease (STD) or becoming pregnant. Indeed, a key concern of health education is to make adolescents aware that there *are* risks associated with many of the behaviors in which they engage. It seems best, then, to employ the term *risk behavior* rather than *risk-taking behavior* and to apply it to any behavior that can compromise adolescent development—whether or not the adolescent is motivated by, or even aware of, the risk involved. Such usage would not only keep the explanation of adolescent risk behavior problematic but encourage the quest for a more general conceptual account.

The Organization of Adolescent Risk Behavior and the Concept of Life-Style

Another issue requires attention as we explore the way toward a general conceptual framework for adolescent risk behavior. This issue is the degree to which there is structure and organization among the different risk behaviors in adolescence. Stated in other terms, the issue is whether there is intraindividual covariation among risk behaviors so that they cluster or form what might be called a risk behavior syndrome. It makes an enormous difference, for both understanding and intervention, to be dealing with separate, independent, and isolated risk behaviors or, instead, with an organized constellation of risk behaviors that are interrelated and covary. The former perspective has sustained what might be called the "problem-of-the-week" approach, in which efforts are mobilized to fight teenage pregnancy one week, drunk driving the next, illicit drug use the next, crime after that, and so on. It is also the perspective that characterizes the separate mission orientations of the various federal agencies, one for alcohol abuse, one for drug abuse, one for mental health, sexual behavior in yet another agency, and delinquency elsewhere. The latter perspective, on the other hand, suggests a more comprehensive and simultaneous concern with the entire array of adolescent risk behaviors and promotes efforts to understand and alter the circumstances that give rise to and sustain such clusters or syndromes of risk behavior in adolescence.

By now, a fair amount of evidence has been accumulated on this question, and there is considerable support for the covariation perspective. The evidence for covariation is strongest for those risk behaviors that are also problem behaviors, for example, drug use, delinquency, alcohol abuse, and sexual precocity. In one of our early longitudinal studies of high school youth, for example, we found that 61 % of marijuana users were sexually experienced compared with only 18 % of nonusers (Jessor & Jessor, 1977). In our later research, using maximum-likelihood factor analysis, we provided additional support for the interrelatedness of adolescent problem behaviors by showing that a single factor accounts for their positive intercorrelations (Donovan & Jessor, 1985; Donovan, Jessor, & Costa, 1988). Further support comes from latent variable analyses of data from our recent study of samples of junior and senior high school youth that include White, Black, and Hispanic adolescents. These analyses show, once again, the interrelatedness of adolescent problem behavior; they also show that a single, second-order latent variable can account for that interrelatedness within all of the ethnic, gender, and school-level subgroups.

The evidence for covariation has been less strong where nonproblem, health-risk behaviors, such as eating, exercise, and safety behaviors, are involved. In the recent study just cited, however, we have been able to show that modest interrelations do obtain among such health behaviors and that, again, a single, second-order latent variable accounts for those relations (Donovan, Jessor, & Costa, 1993). In addition, there are modest negative correlations between the problem behaviors and the health-promoting behaviors. The literature on the entire covariation issue has recently been reviewed in extensive detail (Osgood, 1991; Elliott, 1993).

Overall, the empirical evidence supports the existence of organized patterns of adolescent risk behaviors. These structures of behaviors, taken together, reflect an adolescent's way of being in the world. Their structure or organization raises interesting questions about the origin or source of the covariation and patterning. Part of the answer probably lies in the social ecology of adolescent life, an ecology that provides socially organized opportunities to learn risk behaviors together and normative expectations that they be performed together. Part of the answer probably also lies in the fact that different risk behaviors can serve the same functions: for example, both illicit drug use and precocious sexual activity can provide a way of affirming independence from parents.

The key import of the evidence about covariation among risk behaviors is the support it provides for the organizing concept of life-style. Drawn from the lexicon of common language, the life-style notion has a core meaning denoting an organized pattern of interrelated behaviors. According to one scholar seeking to formalize the term, life-style consists of "expressive [i.e., functional] behaviors… a distinctive and hence recognizable mode of living" (Sobel, 1981). The utility of the concept of life-style, referring as it does to the constellation or syndrome of risk behavior, is that it directs our attention to the adolescent as a whole actor rather than to each of the risk behaviors, one after another. Equally important, it raises a serious question about whether intervention efforts should remain focused, as they have been, on specific behaviors (e.g., illicit drug use) or rather on influencing an adolescent's life-style as a whole.

A General Conceptual Framework for Adolescent Risk Behavior

The discussion to this point has sought to incorporate adolescent behavior into an epidemiological perspective on risk factors. That has involved some reformulation of traditional thinking about risk and about what it is that is at risk, a reformulation hospitable to psychosocial, as well as biomedical outcomes. We have argued that, as risk factors, behaviors such as illicit drug use, school dropout, unprotected sexual intercourse, and delinquency can compromise successful adolescent development and jeopardize the life chances of youth. The focus, thus far, has been on the psychosocial outcomes and consequences of risk factors when they are behaviors. It is now possible to explore behavioral risk factors in the other direction, that is, in terms of their psychosocial antecedents and determinants. Such exploration will lead us to a general conceptual framework for adolescent risk behavior and will illuminate, at the same time, the merging of the epidemiological perspective with that of social/developmental psychology.

The effort to conceptualize and elaborate the antecedents or determinants of risk behaviors, as established risk factors, can continue to use the orientation of epidemiology in the identification of risk factors. Now the key question becomes, What are the risk factors for the (behavioral) risk factors? Or, in the present case, What are the risk factors for the risk behaviors? That epidemiological concern turns out to be identical to the standard concern of social-psychological inquiry, namely, how to explain complex social behavior. In both endeavors, the aim is to move back from identified risk factors to establish what one epidemiologist termed the "web of causation" (MacMahon, Pugh, & Ipsen, 1960), that is, the explanatory framework in which they are embedded and which can provide a logical account of their distribution and occurrence. Indeed, it was another epidemiologist, Milton Terris, who chastised his colleagues for their excessive preoccupation with proximal risk factors—the microorganism in infectious disease, tobacco or salt in chronic disease—while largely ignoring those that are distal: "the whole complex of social and other environmental factors that create that cause, and bring it into effective contact with the host" (Terris, 1983). The web of causation in epidemiology is isomorphic with explanatory theory in social psychology when behaviors are the risk factors at issue.

A comprehensive social-psychological framework for explaining behavior generally includes four major explanatory domains or sources of variance: social environment, perceived environment, personality, and (other) behavior. Although not traditional, more recent explanatory efforts have increasingly sought to engage a fifth domain, namely, biology/genetics. Taken together and fully articulated, these five domains would constitute the "web of causation" or the general explanatory framework for adolescent risk behavior. The schema presented in Fig. 8.1 represents the five domains, illustrates their content, and specifies their relationships to each other, to risk behavior, and to potential outcomes of risk.

Before elaborating on the specific content of the various conceptual domains in the schema, I want to make some general comments about the framework as a whole. First, the framework makes apparent the complexity that is required of any responsible account of adolescent risk behavior. That account would need to engage multiple explanatory domains as well as their interactions; an explanation that confines itself to any single domain—whether genetics, the social environment, or personality—is certain to be incomplete at best and parochial at worst. Further, the widespread proclivity in the field to fasten on single-variable interventions, increasing self-esteem, say, or providing adolescents with mentors, can garner little support from such a framework, given the large array of factors and domains that must be seen to influence risk behavior.

Second, the domains that constitute the web of causation are each represented as having direct effects on adolescent risk behavior. That makes it useful to consider each domain as a separate source of risk—social environment risk, perceived environment risk, personality risk, and so on—and to try to articulate their component variables or determinants or, in epidemiological terms, their risk factors. Third, the various risk domains are also represented as having indirect effects on adolescent risk behavior, effects that are mediated through other risk domains (for reasons of clarity, not all the interconnecting arrows have been drawn). Thus, beyond their direct effects, social environment risk factors, say, poverty and racial/or ethnic discrimination, may influence the risk factor of low perceived life chances in the personality domain and, thereby, indirectly influence risk behavior. Knowledge of direct and indirect effects ought to be of great importance to the design of intervention efforts and to decisions about the most promising loci of intervention.

Fourth, complex as the schema is already, it represents only the structure of risk factors, risk behaviors, and risk outcomes cross-sectionally, that is, at a moment in time. Of fundamental importance, and entirely missing from the figure, are the *changes* going on in each of the domains. Processes of developmental change in the adolescent and of social and historical change in the adolescent's context are, although unrepresented, clearly not meant to be ignored. Fifth, causal influence in the figure needs to be thought of as bidirectional from top to bottom and also from bottom to top. Although the primary concern of this paper has been with providing an account of risk behavior (therefore, a top-to-bottom emphasis), the bidirectional

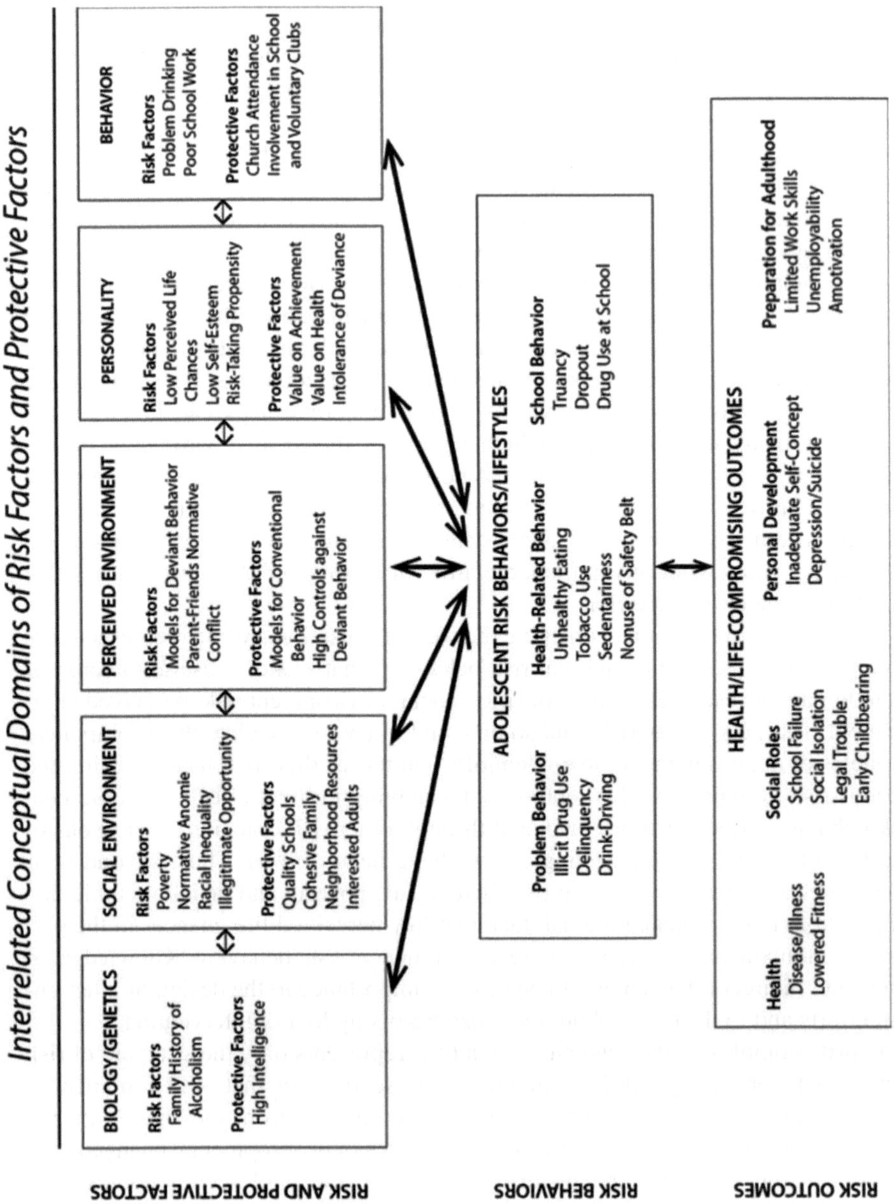

Fig. 8.1 A conceptual framework for adolescent risk behavior: Risk and protective factors, risk behaviors, and risk outcomes

arrows indicate that, of course, engaging in risk behavior can also affect the various domains of risk factors (a bottom-to-top influence). It is this bi- or multidirectionality of the social-psychological framework that makes the web of causation metaphor so apposite.

The particular risk factors that have been listed in each of the different risk domains are, for the most part, drawn from the research literature or implicated in various conceptual analyses of adolescent risk behavior. They are only a selected set, obviously, and meant to be illustrative. Measures of many of the variables, especially those in the perceived environment, the personality, and the behavior domains, have been employed repeatedly in our own work on Problem Behavior Theory, which is a specific variant of the general framework in Fig. 8.1. Multiple regression analyses, employing a dozen or so of the measures, generally yield multiple correlations (*R*s) of about .70 when accounting for an index of multiple-problem behavior among adolescents, and the *R*s range between .50 and .80 when various specific risk behaviors such as problem drinking or illicit drug use are being predicted. Thus, between 25 % and 65 % of the variance in adolescent risk behavior is explained, and close to 50 % is modal (Jessor & Jessor, 1977; Jessor, 1987; Jessor, Donovan, & Costa, 1991). The measures that tend to be invariantly important across our different studies include low expectations for school achievement and low attitudinal intolerance of deviance in the personality domain; models for problem behavior among friends in the perceived environment domain; and marijuana use and poor schoolwork in the behavior domain.

These results, ours and those of many other workers in the field, provide encouraging empirical support for the web of causation shown in Fig. 8.1. At the same time, however, they reveal that a large segment of the variance is left unexplained. In our own work as well as in that of others, I believe this is due, at least in part, to a less than satisfactory grasp on the properties of the social environment, whose ultimate importance cannot be gainsaid. The distribution of a variety of adolescent risk behaviors reflects the circumstances of poverty, racial or ethnic marginality, and limited life chances, as well as the presence of an underground structure of illegitimate opportunity. Such circumstances are not well captured, however, by the usual measures of socioeconomic status, especially for adolescents, and this issue presents a crucial challenge to researchers in this field.

The Role of Protective Factors in Adolescent Risk Behavior

There is a final aspect of the framework shown in Fig. 8.1 that remains to be addressed, namely, the *protective factors* that are listed in each of the risk domains. The conceptual role of protective factors is to help explain a fact that is part of common awareness, namely, that many adolescents who seem to be at high risk nevertheless do not succumb to risk behavior, or are less involved in it than their peers, or, if involved, seem to abandon it more rapidly than others. Stated otherwise, many adolescents growing up under conditions of pervasive adversity, limited resources, and intense pressures toward the transgression of conventional norms manage to overcome such circumstances and to "make it." What enables them to avoid entanglements with the criminal justice system, to remain aloof from antisocial peer groups, to avoid becoming pregnant, to do well in school, to acquire the necessary skills for the transition to work and other adult roles, and to develop a sense of personal adequacy and competence?

One answer to that query would be that, appearances to the contrary notwithstanding, those who make it were, in fact, not really at high risk. For some reason, they were fortunate in not actually being exposed to or experiencing the variety of risk factors that seemed to be part of the context of their lives. In short, they were, somehow, not actually at risk or at as high risk as might have been expected. Although that is conceivable, a more likely answer is that there were indeed exposure to and experience of risk, but that they were countered by exposure to and experience of protection. Protective factors are considered by both Garmezy (1985) and Rutter (1990) to moderate, buffer, insulate against, and, thereby, mitigate the impact of risk on adolescent behavior and development.

It is useful to think of protective factors as operating within each of the conceptual domains: in the social environment, a cohesive family, a neighborhood with informal resources, a caring adult; in the perceived environment, peer models for conventional behavior, and strict social controls; in the personality domain, high value on academic achievement and on health, and high intolerance of deviance; and, in the behavior domain, involvement in conventional behavior, such as church attendance and participation in school activities. To the extent that protective factors such as these are present and operative, they should attenuate, counter, or balance the impact and effects of risk factors.

There is some argument within the field about whether protective factors are merely the opposite or low end of risk factors or are, indeed, different factors that function actively to promote positive behavior and development and, in so doing, have a direct mitigating effect on the impact of risk factors. Heuristically, the latter position seems more useful, and the various factors selected as illustrative of protection in the different risk domains in Fig. 8.1 were chosen to be of that sort. The mitigating role of protection is only demonstrable logically in the presence of risk (Rutter, 1990). In recent analyses of our own data, we classified junior and senior high school males and females, on the basis of a six-component composite-risk factor score, into no risk, moderate risk, and high risk groups. We then cross-classified each risk group into high and low protection subgroups based on a seven-component composite protective factor score. Analysis of variance of involvement in problem behavior showed that high versus low protection made no difference in amount of problem behavior involvement for the no risk groups; it did make a significant difference, however, for both the moderate risk and high risk groups. Those with high protection had significantly lower problem behavior scores than those with low protection, and the interaction was significant. These findings support the logic of protection, and they also illustrate the salutary role that protective factors can play in minimizing the impact of exposure to and experience with risk factors.

Adolescents At Risk: What Does "At Risk" Really Mean?

The conceptual framework can contribute to a more systematic understanding of what is meant when we speak of adolescents being "at risk" or, perhaps more important, being at "high risk." The issue here is how to deal with variation in the magnitude of psychosocial risk.

What is immediately apparent from the conceptual framework is that being at risk can have two quite different meanings. For adolescents already involved in risk behavior, usually those who are older, "at risk" can mean being at risk for health- and life-compromising outcomes: early pregnancy, school failure, trouble with the law, unemployability, inadequate self-concept. The focus here is on the degree of risk associated with the engagement in risk behaviors—illicit drug use, or problem drinking, or cigarette smoking, or precocious sex, or truancy. What is the risk that such engagement will compromise adolescent health, adolescent life, or successful adolescent development? This meaning of being at risk represents a later developmental stage in the ontogeny of risk, a stage wherein risk behaviors are already practiced and intervention is more appropriate than prevention.

For this stage, the assessment of the magnitude of risk would certainly include (1) the intensity of involvement in any particular risk behavior, from a level of exploration to a level of commitment; (2) the number of different risk behaviors an adolescent is involved in and the degree to which they constitute an organized pattern or life-style; (3) the timing of age of onset of the risk behaviors (since evidence links early onset to chronicity and intensity); and (4) the degree of simultaneous involvement in protective behaviors. High risk, at this stage, would imply serious and long-term involvement in an organized pattern of risk behaviors and little involvement in protective behaviors.

For adolescents not yet involved in risk behavior, usually those who are younger, being "at risk" means something else, namely, the risk for initiating, onsetting, or becoming involved in risk behaviors: for beginning sexual intercourse, for onsetting the use of alcohol and illicit drugs, for starting to cut school, for engaging in delinquent acts. The "at risk" focus here is the degree of risk represented in the various conceptual domains of risk in Fig. 8.1 and the likelihood that that risk will generate involvement in risk behaviors. This meaning of being at risk represents an earlier stage in the ontogeny of risk, a stage before risk behaviors have been engaged in, and a stage in which the term *prevention,* or *primary prevention,* seems more appropriate. For this stage, the assessment of the magnitude of risk would require consideration of the following: (1) the number and intensity of risk factors in a particular risk domain, (2) the number and intensity of protective factors in that same domain; (3) the pervasiveness of risk factors across the multiple risk domains, (4) the pervasiveness of protective factors across the multiple domains. To be "at high risk" at this stage would mean that there are multiple and serious risk factors in multiple domains and little in the way of protective factors in those same domains.

A distinction between the two stages of being "at risk" seems useful for both understanding and action; it should not be drawn too sharply, however. The meaning of being at risk sketched out for older adolescents, those already involved in risk behavior, would also need, of course, to consider the degree of risk and of protection in the various conceptual domains in addition to its focus on the extent of their involvement in risk behavior. Whether a risk behavior such as precocious sexual intercourse puts an adolescent at risk for life-compromising outcomes such as early pregnancy and unemployability is undoubtedly influenced by the risk factors and protective factors in that adolescent's social environment. Remaining in school or returning to school may well hinge on the availability of social support, resources for child care, presence of a caring adult, and so forth, in that environment. In short, risk for health- and life-compromising outcomes should be seen as "nested" in the conceptual framework, with the risk from risk behaviors nested in the risk from the various conceptual domains.

A final point needs to be made in considering the appraisal of variation in magnitude of risk, one that has been assumed in the discussion but not stated explicitly. Degree of risk needs to be treated conceptually as a resultant, an outcome of the balance of risk and protection. Two adolescents characterized by the same pattern of risk factors may be at very different degrees of risk, depending on the protective factors that affect their lives. The logic of the conceptual framework requires arriving at a resultant that reflects the balance of risk and protection. An assessment of risk that ignores protection can turn out to be severely off the mark.

Implications for Prevention/Intervention

First, and perhaps of overriding importance, is the import of the complexity of the web of causation that has been proposed. What that complexity suggests is that prevention and intervention efforts that are comprehensive promise to yield greater success than those that are more limited in scope. Programs that fail to engage multiple risk domains are unlikely to be successful or to generate lasting effects. Second, programs need to design efforts that can simultaneously reduce risk and promote protection; neither strategy alone would seem optimal for effecting change. Third, programs directed at the organization and patterning of multiple risk behaviors may be more appropriate than programs focused on specific behaviors alone. Life-style change, although obviously a challenge, has the promise of more pervasive and more enduring impact on the repertoire of risk behaviors. Fourth, programs that acknowledge the salience of the social environment would seem especially critical. Young people growing up in adverse social environments are in double jeopardy: not only are risk factors more intense and more prevalent in such contexts but protective factors are less available if not, indeed, absent for many. It is in contexts such as these that risk behaviors are more likely to have irretrievable outcomes, whereas the very same behaviors in a less adverse setting often gain for the adolescent a "second chance," that is, the opportunity and support for getting back on track. Finally, the emphasis on risk behavior and on life-style should not be translated into making individuals alone responsible for removing the risk in their lives; such an approach would tend to "blame the victim." The present conceptual framework makes it patently clear that risk is embedded in the larger social context of adolescent life and that reduction in risk requires social change as well.

Conclusion

This presentation has sought to examine how the confluence of epidemiology and social psychology can illuminate an important social problem, adolescent risk behavior. The conceptual framework that has been elaborated is an effort to represent both social-psychological and behavioral epidemiology theory. The epidemiologist Reuel Stallones speaks of "a territory of especial beauty at the intersection of the biomedical and social sciences" (Stallones, 1980). It was the attractiveness of that territory for understanding complex human behavior that motivated this effort; hopefully its attractiveness will draw other scientists and practitioners to explore the same terrain.

I began this discussion with a brief prolegomenon, and I cannot in good conscience resist a brief afterword. It seems to me that the kind of analysis presented here and our shared awareness of the worsening plight of young people growing up poor in our society demand something more from us than collegial and scholarly interchange. Milton Terris has pointed out that issues such as those dealt with in this paper "have become basic questions of economic and social policy… [and they bring us] into direct confrontation with some of the most powerful economic and political forces in the nation" (Terris, 1983). A government that was able to find the needed resources for military adventures in Southeast Asia, in Central America, and now in the Middle East surely can find them for its own youth in its decaying cities and on its impoverished farms. Perhaps we also need to consider how to make that happen.

Acknowledgments I am indebted to Drs. John E. Donovan and Frances Costa, who have been my colleagues in the research that has shaped some of the ideas in this paper. The support of the W. T. Grant Foundation (Grant No. 88119488) for research on adolescent health behaviors is gratefully acknowledged. My experience on the Carnegie Council on Adolescent Development and my role in the MacArthur Foundation's Research Program on Successful Adolescent Development among Youth in High-Risk Settings have helped me to think more deeply about some of the issues addressed here.

References

Donovan, J. E., & Jessor, R. (1985). Structure of problem behavior in adolescence and young adulthood. *Journal of Consulting and Clinical Psychology, 53*(6), 890–904.

Donovan, J. E., Jessor, R., & Costa, F. M. (1988). Syndrome of problem behavior in adolescence: A replication. *Journal of Consulting and Clinical Psychology, 56*(5), 762–765.

Donovan, J. E., Jessor, R., & Costa, F. M. (1993). Structure of health-enhancing behavior in adolescence: A latent-variable approach. *Journal of Health and Social Behavior, 34*(4), 346–362.

Elliott, D. S. (1993). Health-enhancing and health-compromising lifestyles. In S. G. Millstein, A. C. Petersen, & E. O. Nightingale (Eds.), *Promoting the health of adolescents: New directions for the twenty-first century* (pp. 119–150). New York: Oxford University Press.

Garmezy, N. (1985). Stress-resistant children: The search for protective factors. In J. E. Stevenson (Ed.), *Recent research in developmental psychopathology* (pp. 213–233). Oxford: Pergamon Press.

Jessor, R. (1987). Problem Behavior Theory, psychosocial development, and adolescent problem drinking. *British Journal of Addiction, 82*(4), 331–342.

Jessor, R., Donovan, J. E., & Costa, F. M. (1991). *Beyond adolescence: Problem behavior and young adult development*. New York: Cambridge University Press.

Jessor, R., & Jessor, S. L. (1977). *Problem behavior and psychosocial development: A longitudinal study of youth*. New York: Academic Press.

MacMahon, B., Pugh, T. F., & Ipsen, J. (1960). *Epidemiologic methods*. Boston: Little, Brown.

Osgood, D. W. (1991). *Covariation among health problems in adolescence*. Washington, DC: Office of Technology Assessment.

Rutter, M. (1990). Psychosocial resilience and protective mechanisms. In J. Rolf, A. S. Masten, D. Cicchetti, K. H. Nuechterlein, & S. Weintraub (Eds.), *Risk and protective factors in the development of psychopathology* (pp. 181–214). Cambridge: Cambridge University Press.

Sobel, M. E. (1981). *Lifestyle and social structure: Concepts, definitions, analyses*. New York: Academic Press.

Stallones, R. A. (1980). To advance epidemiology. *Annual Review of Public Health, 1*, 69–82.

Terris, M. (1983). The complex tasks of the second epidemiologic revolution: The Joseph W. Mountin lecture. *Journal of Public Health Policy, 4*(1), 8–24.

Chapter 9
Problem Behavior Theory and the Dynamics of Protection and Risk

Richard Jessor, Jill Van Den Bos, Judith Vanderryn, Frances M. Costa, and Mark S. Turbin

Research on adolescent involvement in problem behavior, indeed, on adolescent behavior and development more generally, has become more complex in recent years. Multivariate inquiries now map both social and personal influences over time and are displacing single-variable, single-domain, cross-sectional approaches (Jessor, 1993). Increased complexity is also evident in studies that go beyond traditional concerns with demonstrating "main effects" to explore interactive relations among predictor variables as well, and to examine whether those interactions moderate predicted linkages with behavior. The latter kind of complexity is the focus of this article. We report an investigation of the relationships between psychosocial protective factors and involvement in problem behavior in adolescence: alcohol and drug use, delinquency, and sexual precocity. The effects of protective factors and their role as moderators of the relationship between risk factors and problem behavior are examined cross-sectionally as well as over time.

Reprinted with permission from:
Jessor, R., Van Den Bos, J., Vanderryn, J., Costa, F. M., & Turbin, M. S. (1995). Protective factors in adolescent problem behavior: Moderator effects and developmental change. *Developmental Psychology, 31*(6), 923–933.

R. Jessor (✉)
Institute of Behavioral Science, University of Colorado at Boulder, Boulder, CO, USA
e-mail: jessor@Colorado.edu

J. Van Den Bos
Milliman Company, Denver, CO, USA

J. Vanderryn
Mountain View TLC, Durango, CO, USA

F.M. Costa
University of Colorado Boulder, Boulder, CO, USA

M.S. Turbin
Kalispell, MT, USA

R. Jessor, *The Origins and Development of Problem Behavior Theory*,
Advancing Responsible Adolescent Development,
DOI 10.1007/978-3-319-40886-6_9

Interest in protective factors emerged initially from work in developmental psychopathology. The observation, among children similarly exposed to risk for psychopathology, that many nevertheless escaped its impact or consequences led Garmezy and others (Garmezy, 1985; Garmezy & Masten, 1986; Rutter, 1987; Werner, 1989a, 1989b) to articulate variables that might be protective, that is, that might serve to moderate, buffer, or insulate against risk. Variation in risk alone had preoccupied previous researchers, but the new attention to protective factors provided a basis for investigators to account for individual differences in outcome in which exposure to risk was essentially held constant. More recently, the possibility of protective factors mitigating the impact of risk has been extended beyond psychopathology to involvement in adolescent drug and alcohol use (Brook, Whiteman, Cohen, & Tanaka, 1992; Felix-Ortiz & Newcomb, 1992; Hawkins, Catalano, & Miller, 1992; Stacy, Newcomb, & Bentler, 1992; Stacy, Sussman, Dent, Burton, & Flay, 1992; Wills, Vaccaro, & McNamara, 1992).

Although the concept of risk, borrowed largely from epidemiology, is widely understood, the same is not true for protection. Risk factors are those conditions or variables that are associated with a higher likelihood of negative or undesirable outcomes—morbidity or mortality, in classical usage, or, more recently, behaviors that can compromise health, well-being, or social performance. There has been far less consensus about the concept and operationalization of protective factors. Protection has sometimes been defined simply as the absence of risk or as the low end of a risk variable. Rutter (1987) argued most forcefully, however, that protective factors and risk factors should be treated as conceptually distinct rather than as opposite ends of a single dimension, and that view is now coming to be shared by most others (Felix-Ortiz & Newcomb, 1992; Hawkins et al., 1992; Jessor, 1991; Luthar & Zigler, 1991; Pellegrini, 1990). In this latter perspective, protective factors are considered independent variables that can have their own direct effects on behavior but that, in addition, can moderate the relation between risk factors and behavior.

Protective factors are conceptualized as decreasing the likelihood of engaging in problem behavior: through direct personal or social controls against its occurrence (e.g., strong religious commitment or predictable parental sanctions); through involvement in activities that tend to be incompatible with or alternatives to problem behavior (e.g., activities with the family or with church groups); and through orientations toward and commitments to conventional institutions (e.g., schools) or to adult society more generally. In contrast, risk factors are conceptualized as increasing the likelihood of engaging in problem behavior: through direct instigation or encouragement (e.g., failure or frustration instigating a coping response, or models and influence from peers); through increased vulnerability for normative transgression (e.g., low self-esteem); and through greater opportunity to engage in problem behavior (e.g., membership in an antisocial peer group).

Research on risk and protective factors has often shown them to be negatively related, but that relationship ought not to be seen as a logical necessity. Rather, it may simply reflect a particular history of personal experience or a particular organization of the social ecology; for example, in those contexts in which protection is high, risk is usually low, and vice versa. These empirical relations notwithstanding, it remains logically possible, for example, to find high risk accompanied by high protection, rather than high risk necessarily implying low protection. An adolescent may well have antisocial friends and yet be committed to and involved in school. Although risk and protection may be inversely related empirically, the conceptual perspective is that they are best treated as orthogonal.

As already noted, the influence of protective factors, whether in relation to substance use or to any other adolescent problem behavior, is to lessen the likelihood of its occurrence. When protective factors serve, in addition, as moderators, they modify the relation between risk and problem behavior: That relationship, linear and positive when protection is low or absent, is markedly attenuated when protection is high. This description of a differential relation of risk to problem behavior at different levels of protection is another way of specifying an interaction between risk and protection in their relation to adolescent involvement in problem behavior.

A large number of protective factors, ecological as well as personal, have been explored as moderators of the relationship of risk to behavioral outcomes. Garmezy (1985) organized protection variables into three categories: (a) dispositional attributes, that is, individual differences, such as high self-efficacy; (b) family attributes, such as parental support and affection; and (c) extrafamilial circumstances, such as support from other adults, or strong community integration. In research on alcohol and drug use, the protective factors studied have ranged from bonding to conventional society (Hawkins et al., 1992) to supportive relations with parents (Felix-Ortiz & Newcomb, 1992; Wills et al., 1992) to high religiosity and law abidance (Felix-Ortiz & Newcomb, 1992; Stacy, Newcomb, & Bentler, et al., 1992) to self-efficacy in social relations (Stacy, Sussman, et al., 1992).

Our own approach to the delineation of protective factors in adolescence has relied on the systematic implications of Problem Behavior Theory (Jessor, Donovan, & Costa, 1991; Jessor, Graves, Hanson, & Jessor, 1968; Jessor & Jessor, 1977). In each of the three psychosocial explanatory systems in the theory—the personality system, the perceived environment system, and the behavior system—the variables are specified either as instigators to or controls against involvement in problem behavior. Instigations are analogous to risk factors, and controls are analogous to protective factors. Although the risk and protective factors used in this study originate from a particular theory, their commonality with the variables used by others, as noted earlier, will be obvious.

Seven protective variables were used in the present research: (a) positive orientation to school, (b) positive orientation to health, and (c) intolerant attitudes toward deviance (and, in later waves, religiosity) from the personality system; (d) positive relations with adults, (e) the perception of strong social controls or sanctions for transgression, and (f) awareness of friends who model conventional behavior, from the perceived environment system; and (g) actual involvement in prosocial behaviors, such as volunteer work and family activities, from the behavior system. Six risk variables were used: (a) low expectations for success, (b) low self-esteem, and (c) a general sense of hopelessness about life, from the personality system; (d) awareness of friends who model involvement in problem behavior and (e) a greater orientation toward friends than toward parents, from the perceived environment system; and (f) poor school achievement (and, in later waves, school dropout), from the behavior system. The measurement of each of these variables and its rationale as a risk or protective factor are elaborated in the Method section.

In research in which multiple risk factors and multiple protective factors have been assessed, there has been growing interest in the amount of risk or the amount of protection as a key parameter, as well as in the various types of risk or protection represented by the specific measures. Findings have shown substantial linear relations between the number of different risk factors and a variety of outcomes (Bry, 1983; Garmezy, 1985; Jessor et al., 1968, Chap. 11; Newcomb, Maddahian, & Bentler, 1986; Sameroff, Seifer, Baldwin, & Baldwin, 1993; Sameroff, Seifer, Barocas, Zax, & Greenspan, 1987; Small & Luster, 1994; Werner, 1989a, 1989b). Rutter (1979) also advocated counting the number of risk (and protective) factors because he found that different risk factors potentiated each other. A counting or cumulative approach to risk and protective factors focuses on variation in the number of different risk or protective factors involved. Exploring this approach is a salient concern of the present investigation, although we also examine the role of particular risk and protective factors.

Unlike earlier research on the moderating role of protective factors, in which the concern was with psychopathology or, more recently, with substance use, the focus of the present study is on the larger domain of adolescent problem behavior, including problem drinking, illicit drug use, delinquent behavior and early sexual intercourse. The aim of the present research is to explore the role of psychosocial protective factors in adolescent problem behavior. Our first concern is to determine whether protective factors are, indeed, associated with lower levels of involvement in problem behavior. Our second concern is to determine whether protective factors moderate the relationship between risk and problem behavior involvement. And our third concern is to determine whether protective factors are related to change in adolescent problem behavior over subsequent time.

Method

Study Design and Procedure

The data used in this article were collected as part of a longitudinal study of problem behavior and health-related behavior in adolescence. Begun in the spring of 1989, the study has involved four annual waves of data collection on middle school and high school youths. Participants were in Grades 7 to 9 at Wave 1 when data were collected in six middle schools and four high schools in a large metropolitan school district in the Rocky Mountain region. Participating schools were chosen for the study by the school district administration to maximize representation of Hispanic and Black students from inner-city areas.

Active parental and personal consent was sought for all students enrolled in the selected schools. Letters describing the study were written to the parents and the students, and signed consent forms were returned to the school. All of the letters and consent forms were written in both English and Spanish. Study participants were released from class to take part in large-group administration sessions. Bilingual versions of the questionnaire were available for those students who preferred to work in Spanish. Each student received a token payment of $5 for each wave.

Participants

A total of 2410 students in Grades 7, 8, and 9 participated in the first wave of the study in 1989. Although participation rates varied from school to school, questionnaires were filled out by 67 % of the middle school students (Grades 7 and 8) and by 49 % of the high school students (Grade 9). The less-than-desirable initial participation rate was due largely to the necessity of obtaining active parental consent and to the difficulty of eliciting a response from many of the parents. Comparisons of the Wave-1 participants with nonparticipants, using school record data, show that the participant sample did represent the full range of scores on grade point average, standardized achievement test scores, disciplinary actions, and school absences, although participants were, on the average, more conventional than nonparticipants on these indicators.

At the Wave-2 (1990) data collection, questionnaires were completed by 2016 students, or 84 % of the Wave-1 sample. At Wave 3 (1991), 1974 students (82 % of the Wave-1 sample) filled out questionnaires, and, in Wave 4, 1782 students (74 % of the Wave-1 sample) took part. Overall, 1591 students filled out all four annual questionnaires; they represent 66 % of the Wave-1 sample. The effect of the attrition of 819 participants, after Wave 1, was examined. (The non-four-wave participants included participants having only one [$n=212$], two [$n=215$], or three [$n=392$] waves of data.) Their Wave-1 mean scores on 12 selected measures from the questionnaire were compared with the Wave-1 mean scores of the 1591 four-wave participants on those same measures. The attrition subsample was less conventional or more problem-prone on 9 of the measures, and there was no difference on 3 of the measures. Despite those mean differences, the intercorrelations among the measures were similar in both groups. A test of the equality of the covariance structure matrices in the two groups, based on nine representative variables, yielded a goodness-of-fit index of .997. Although the chi-square of 79.8 was significant ($p<.001$), it was only slightly more than twice the 36 degrees of freedom. Thus, despite the bias toward greater conventionality in the participating four-wave sample, relations among their measures would not be very different had the attrition not occurred.

Forty-three percent of the four-wave longitudinal sample are male, and equal proportions of the sample are in the 7th-, 8th-, and 9th-grade starting cohorts. With respect to race/ethnicity, 36 % of the sample are White, 36 % Hispanic, 22 % Black, 4 % Asian, and 2 % Native American. Forty-five percent of the participants are from intact families; 22 % have a stepparent living with them (usually stepfather); 29 % live with one parent (usually mother); and 3 % live with other relatives or guardians. The analyses presented in this article were carried out using data from all the White, Hispanic, and Black participants with four complete waves of data ($N=1486$).

Measurement of Risk and Protection

Six measures of risk and 7 measures of protection were obtained from the Wave-1 (1989) data, and they are used as continuous variables in later multivariate analyses of problem behavior involvement. To establish an index of the number of risk factors and protective factors, however, we dichotomized scores on each measure to represent the presence or absence of that risk factor or protective factor using the procedure described later. An overall Risk Factor Index (RFI) and an overall Protective Factor Index (PR) were then developed on the basis of summative scores that characterized each participant. Dichotomization of scores on each of the individual measures of risk or protection was done so as to yield roughly the extreme 30 % of participants on that measure, thus maximizing the likelihood that the risk factor or the protective factor was indeed present. An extreme score on a measure was assigned the value of 1, indicating the presence of risk or of protection on the different measures. A score of 0 indicates no risk or no protection on the respective measures.

Measures of protection. Three protective factors represent the personality system. Positive Orientation To School is a nine-item scale measuring attitudes toward school (e.g., "How do you feel about going to school?") and personal value on academic achievement (α=.79). Having a positive orientation toward school constitutes protection against involvement in problem behavior because it reflects positive engagement with a conventional social institution and commitment to its goals. Such an orientation toward conventionality is not compatible with engaging in behaviors that are considered inappropriate by adults and that may also jeopardize school achievement. Positive Orientation Toward Health is a two-component index based on the standardized score on a 7-item scale of personal value on health (α=.67) added to the standardized score on a 10-item scale of personal beliefs about the health consequences of various behaviors such as smoking and eating junk food (α=.76). A positive orientation toward health constitutes protection because it represents a personal control against involvement in behaviors, such as substance use, that can be damaging to or incompatible with health. Attitudinal Intolerance of Deviance is a 10-item attitude scale assessing the judged "wrongness" of certain delinquent- type behaviors, including physical aggression, theft, and property damage (α=.90). Intolerance of deviance constitutes protection because it reflects a commitment to conventional values and disapproval of norm-violative activities, and it serves as a direct personal control against involvement in such activities. Protection in the personality system is thus indicated by a positive orientation toward school, a positive orientation toward health, and high intolerance of deviance.

Three protective factors represent the perceived environment system. Positive Relations With Adults was measured by four questions assessing a respondent's relationships with parents and other adults, including the extent to which parents show interest in the respondent and whether the respondent is able to discuss personal problems with an adult (α=.61). More positive relations with adults constitute protection because adults provide support for conventional behavior and sanctions against problem behavior. Perceived Regulatory Controls was measured by a two-component index based on the standardized score on a seven-item scale assessing the presence of family rules about getting homework done, dating, curfew, doing chores, and so on (α=.57), added to the score on one question about expected sanctions from friends for involvement in deviant behavior. Perception of greater regulatory controls in the social environment constitutes protection because it increases the likelihood that the adolescent will be deterred from problem behaviors, and it helps make clear the types of behavior that are unacceptable to others. Friends Models for Conventional Behavior, a four-item scale assessing the proportion of friends who are in school clubs, attend religious services, are in community or church youth groups, and get good grades in school ($\alpha=.75$), constitutes protection because it reflects greater involvement with conventional peers and more time spent in conventional activities. Protection in the perceived social environment is thus indicated by positive relations with adults, high regulatory controls, and high friends models for conventional behavior.

One measure of protection represents the behavior system. Prosocial Activities is a three-item index that combines involvement and time spent in family activities, in volunteer activities, and in school clubs other than sports. High involvement in prosocial activities constitutes protection because prosocial activities preempt time to become involved in problem behavior and also promote orientations and social networks incompatible with the latter.

The operationalization of protection is thus based on answers to the questionnaire that yield characterizations of the respondent, of the social environment as perceived by the respondent, and of the respondent's behavior.

Measures of risk. Three risk factors represent the personality system. Expectations for Success is a two-component index consisting of the standardized score on a four-item scale of expectations for academic achievement ($\alpha=.85$) added to the standardized score on a nine-item scale of perceived life chances in the opportunity structure ($\alpha=.90$). Together, these components assess anticipated positive life outcomes in various areas such as school, family life, employment, friendships, finances, and so on. Low expectation of achieving these valued life goals constitutes risk for involvement in problem behavior because it can serve to pressure an adolescent toward alternative means, such as substance use or delinquency, to achieve some of those same goals. Self-Esteem is a six-item scale measuring participants' beliefs about their abilities and attributes in various domains, including social skills, academic competence, and personal attractiveness ($\alpha=.66$). A low sense of self-worth and low confidence in one's ability to handle challenges and responsibilities constitute risk because engaging in problem behavior can be a way to cope with such negative feelings. Hopelessness is a two-component index consisting of the standardized score on a four- item scale of depression ($\alpha=.85$) added to the standardized score on a four-item scale of alienation ($\alpha=.67$). Together, these components assess feelings of depression, anxiety, hopelessness, and social alienation. Disengagement from societal norms and feeling isolated from others constitute risk because the social influences that usually serve as controls against engaging in problem behavior are attenuated, and the sense of vulnerability may lead to coping through problem behavior. Risk in the personality system is thus indicated by low expectations for success, low self-esteem, and high hopelessness.

Two risk factors represent the perceived environment system. Friends Models for Problem Behavior is a four-item scale assessing perceived models among friends for cigarette smoking, alcohol use, marijuana use, and sexual intercourse ($\alpha=.75$).

Exposure to friends who model involvement in problem behavior constitutes risk because models (a) provide an opportunity to learn how to engage in the behavior, (b) offer access to supplies that may be necessary for carrying out the behavior, such as cigarettes, alcohol, or other drugs, and (c) indicate that problem behavior is characteristic of the peer group. The Friend Orientation Index is a two-component measure based on standardized scores on two three-item scales, one measuring perceived agreement or compatibility between parents and friends (α=.71) and the other measuring the relative influence of parents and friends on the respondent's outlook, life choices, and behavior (α=.56). Lower parents-friends agreement and higher friends'-relative-to-parents' influence both indicate greater orientation to friends and constitute risk because parents represent and exercise controls against deviant or norm-violative behavior and generally serve as models for conventional values, attitudes, and activities. Risk in the perceived environment system is thus indicated by high friends models for problem behavior and high orientation to friends relative to parents.

One measure of risk, School Record Grade Point Average, represents the behavior system. Grade point averages in the bottom 28 % of the distribution were considered a risk factor. Low school achievement constitutes risk because it may reflect detachment from school, may lower expectations for success in other life areas such as work, may have a negative impact on self-esteem, and may contribute to a sense of personal hopelessness.

Establishing the RFI and the PFI

The RFI and the PFI were computed by adding the dichotomized scores (0 to 1) on the six risk and the seven protective measures, respectively. Scores on the RFI could range from 0 to 6, and scores on the PFI could range from 0 to 7. For respondents missing scores on measures in an index, the missing values were replaced with the mean of the scores for the relevant gender, cohort, and race/ethnicity subgroup.

The RFI and the PFI are summative indexes rather than scales and, as such, would not be expected to show high alpha reliabilities. The RFI had an alpha reliability of .54; the mean inter-item correlation was .16. The PFI had an alpha reliability of .59; the mean inter-item correlation was .17. Corrected item-total correlations for both indexes ranged from .15 to .41. Given the widely varied content of the indexes, these psychometric properties indicated a reasonable degree of internal coherence for both of them.

The Pearson correlation of −.42 (−.39 for the male and −.46 for the female participants) between the RFI and the PFI was in the expected negative direction. The magnitude of this correlation indicated that the two measures, although empirically related as might be expected, shared only a modest proportion of variance and reflected relatively distinct constructs. The magnitude of this correlation between the measures of risk and protection was, incidentally, quite similar to that found in two other recent studies, namely, −.35 in both Wills et al. (1992) and Felix-Ortiz and Newcomb (1992).

Female students had a slightly higher mean score on the RFI than did male students (1.8 vs. 1.6), $F(1, 1484)=8.0$, $p<.01$, and also on the PFI (2.2 vs. 1.8), $F(1, 1484)=21.7$, $p<.001$. Mean scores on the RFI were highest for Hispanics (2.1), followed by Blacks (1.7) and Whites (1.3), $F(2, 1483)=33.7$, $p<.001$. Mean scores on the PFI were highest for Blacks (2.4), followed by Whites (2.1) and Hispanics (1.8), $F(2, 1483)=15.4$, $p<.001$. Cohort scores on the RFI showed an increase in mean as age increased: 1.5, 1.7, and 2.0 for the 7th, 8th, and 9th graders, respectively, $F(2, 1483)=15.1$, $p<.001$. Mean scores on the PFI decreased, but not significantly, after 7th grade: 2.2, 2.0, and 2.0 for 7th, 8th, and 9th graders, respectively.

Measurement of Problem Behavior

The Multiple Problem Behavior Index (MPBI) assesses four different areas of adolescent problem behavior: (a) problem drinking (score range=3–24), based on reports of frequency of drunkenness, frequency of high volume drinking (5 or more drinks per occasion), and negative consequences of drinking ($\alpha=.81$); (b) delinquent-type behavior (score range=10–50), including self-reports of physical aggression, vandalism, theft, and lying ($\alpha=.85$); (c) marijuana involvement (score range=0–8), as reflected in reports of whether the adolescents ever use, frequency of use, availability of marijuana, and the number of times the adolescents have been high ($\alpha=.71$); and (d) sexual intercourse experience (score range=1–2), based on respondents' reports of whether they had ever had sexual intercourse.[1] Measures of the four components of the index were transformed into *T* scores (mean of 50 and standard deviation of 10) and summed.[2]

Male students had a significantly higher MPBI mean score than did female students (202.4 vs. 198.1), $F(1,1484)=7.4$, $p<.01$; mean MPBI score for Hispanics was highest (206.6), followed by Blacks (196.9) and Whites (194.9), $F(1, 1483)=24.6$, $p<.001$; and mean scores across cohorts increased from 191.2 to 200.7 to 208.4 for the 7th-, 8th-, and 9th-grade cohorts, respectively, $F(1, 1483)=42.9$, $p<.001$. The MPBI has an alpha of .75; it has been well established as an important criterion measure in considerable previous work (Jessor & Jessor, 1977).

[1] Mean scores are 4.40 for the problem drinking measure, 16.27 for delinquent-type behavior, 1.68 for marijuana involvement, and 1.22 for sexual intercourse experience. Intercorrelations among these measures are as follows: problem drinking correlates .50, .59, and .34 with delinquent-type behavior, marijuana involvement, and sexual intercourse experience, respectively; delinquent-type behavior correlates .51 and .28 with marijuana involvement and sexual intercourse experience, respectively; and the latter two measures correlate .34. All correlations are significant at $<.001$.

[2] In the Wave-1 data, eight outlying high scores on the MPBI were recoded to approximately three standard deviations above the mean, thereby ensuring a less skewed distribution for the analyses presented in this article.

Analytic Procedures

Hierarchical multiple regression was used in both cross-sectional and longitudinal analyses to assess, first, whether protection is related to adolescent involvement in problem behavior; second, whether protection moderates the relationship between risk and problem behavior involvement; and third, whether protection is related to change in adolescent problem behavior involvement over time.[3]

The demonstration of a moderator effect for protection requires the demonstration of a significant Risk by Protection interaction. Multiple regression provides for the statistical testing of a moderator effect for continuous variables (here the RFI and the PFI) by including their product or interaction term at a later step in the regression equation (Baron & Kenny, 1986; Cohen, 1978; Saunders, 1956). A hierarchical, incremental *F*-test then shows whether the product term, the interaction, adds predictability over and above the account provided by the additive model using just the two predictors.

Results

The Results section is organized into two parts. The first part is based on cross-sectional data from Wave 1 (1989) and examines whether protective factors are related to adolescent involvement in problem behavior and, in addition, whether they moderate the relationship between risk factors and problem behavior involvement. The second part examines whether antecedent protection is related to change in adolescent involvement in problem behavior over time, using the longitudinal data on later problem behavior involvement in Waves 2 (1990), 3 (1991), and 4 (1992).

Cross-Sectional Analyses of Protection and Problem Behavior

We ran hierarchical multiple regression analyses to predict the Wave-1 criterion measure of adolescent involvement in problem behavior, the MPBI. A set of five demographic control measures—gender, two ethnic status dummy variables (White vs. Minority; Hispanic vs. Black), family socioeconomic status (SES), and grade in school (cohort)—was entered in Step 1. In Steps 2 and 3, respectively, the RFI and

---

[3]Five demographic variables are included in all these analyses as control measures: gender, two indicators of race/ethnicity, an index of socioeconomic status, and cohort. The first ethnicity variable contrasts Whites with Hispanics and Blacks, and the second ethnicity variable contrasts Hispanics with Blacks. The SES index is a three-item measure combining participant's reports of mother's and father's educational attainment and father's occupation ($\alpha = .82$). If any of the components of this measure were missing, the remaining information was used alone. Cohort refers to Wave-1 grade in school: Grade 7, 8, or 9.

Table 9.1 Cross-sectional hierarchical regression analysis of the Risk Factor and Protective Factor Indexes With the Multiple Problem Behavior Index: Wave 1 (1989)

Step/predictor measures	β at final step[a]	R^2	R^2 change
1. Demographic Controls		.10***	
Gender	–4.86***		
White or Minority	−1.21*		
Hispanic or Black	2.53**		
Socioeconomic Status	–.08		
Cohort	6.56***		
2. Add Risk Factor Index	7.96***	.23***	.132***
3. Add Protective Factor Index	−1.25*	.24***	.013***
4. Add Risk × Protection Interaction	–.85**	.25***	.004**

[a]Unstandardized regression coefficients are reported because standardized coefficients are inappropriate with interaction terms (see Aiken & West, 1991, pp. 40–47)
*$p \leq .05$. ** $p \leq .01$. *** $p \leq .001$

the PFI were entered. Finally, in Step 4, the cross-product, RFI by PFI, was entered as the interaction term. A significant increase in the multiple R^2 following the entry of the interaction term into a regression analysis already containing the RFI and PFI predictors provides evidence for a moderator effect (see Cohen & Cohen, 1983, pp. 320–324). Results of the hierarchical regression analyses are shown in Table 9.1.

The demographic control measures entered in Step 1 account for a significant portion of the variance in adolescent problem behavior; the R^2 with the MPBI is .10. With the entry of the RFI in Step 2, there is a substantial and significant increment in the amount of variance explained; the R^2 now reaches .23, and the R^2 change of .132 is also highly significant. When the PFI is entered in Step 3, the R^2 increases to .24. The .013 increment is significant and indicates that the PFI accounts for unique variance in the MPBI score in addition to the variance it shares with the RFI, the latter already having been entered. As the unstandardized regression coefficients show, both the RFI (7.96) and the PFI (−1.25) are significantly related to variation in adolescent problem behavior in the direction expected. The data, thus far, provide support for the effect of protection: The higher the number of protective factors, the lower the involvement in problem behavior. The data also support the wealth of previous findings about the effect of risk: The higher the number of risk factors, the greater the involvement in problem behavior.

When the interaction term, RFI by PFI, is added in Step 4, the R^2 change of .004 is also statistically significant. Thus, controlling for sociodemographic factors, and taking into account the effects of the RFI and the PFI, there is still a significant increment in the prediction of problem behavior contributed by the Risk by Protection interaction. This finding provides empirical support for the moderating effect of protection on the relationship between risk and problem behavior in adolescence. The significant regression coefficient of −.85 for the interaction term indicates that the effect of protection is to lessen the impact of risk more when protection is high than when protection is low or absent.

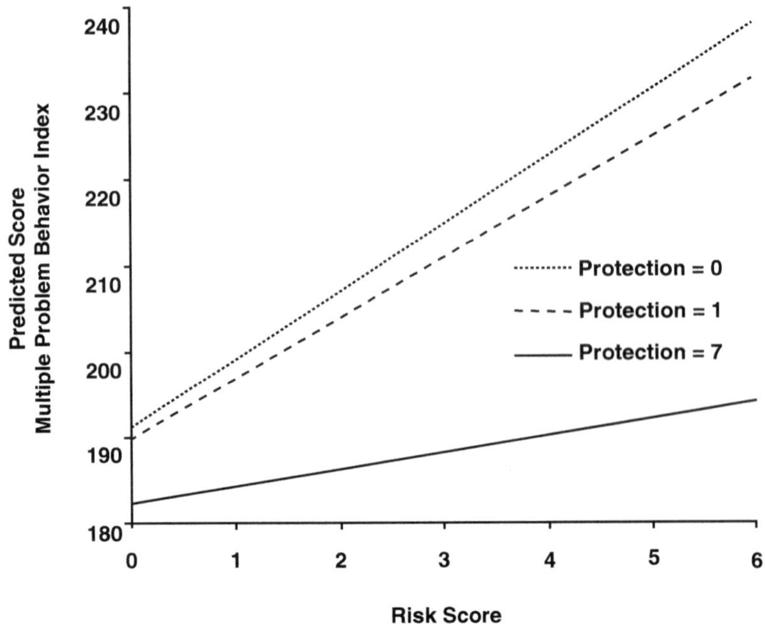

Fig. 9.1 The moderator effect of protection on the relationship of risk to problem behavior: predicted curves

The moderator effect of protection on the relationship between risk and involvement in problem behavior is illustrated in Fig. 9.1. Using the regression analysis findings reported in Table 9.1, we plotted the predicted values of the MPBI score, for different levels of protection, against the level of risk. The ordinate in Fig. 9.1 represents the predicted degree of involvement in problem behavior (the predicted MPBI score); the abscissa represents degree of risk (the RFI score); and the three regression lines represent three different levels of protection from highest protection (PFI score = 7) to lowest protection (PFI score = 1) to an absence of protection (PFI score = 0). The interaction effect is evident. When protection is absent (PFI score = 0), increasing the level of risk shows the largest effect, as illustrated by the steep slope of the regression line. At the minimal level of protection (PFI score = 1), the slope of the regression line is slightly less steep. It is when protection is high (PFI score = 7) that it has a pronounced effect: Increasing the level of risk now makes only a modest difference, that is, the slope of the regression line is relatively shallow. High risk is associated with high involvement in problem behavior when protection is absent or low but not when protection is high. In fact, under the condition of highest protection, the predicted MPBI score for high risk is not much higher than the predicted scores for low risk.

The curves in Fig. 9.1 are predicted from the regression equation represented in Table 9.1; it is also possible to illustrate the moderator role of protection by plotting curves from the actual data. Both the RFI and the PFI were dichotomized as close to the median as possible—at 0 or 1 versus 2 or more—and the significant

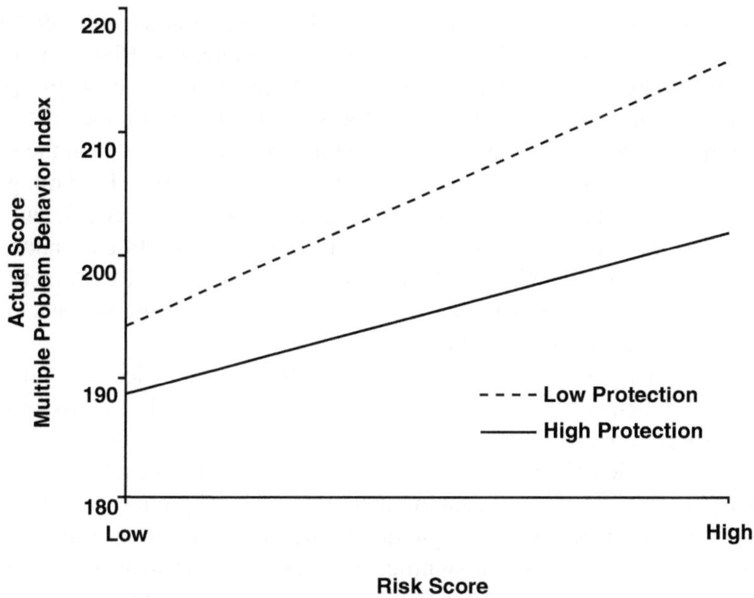

Fig. 9.2 The moderator effect of protection on the relationship of risk to problem behavior: actual curves

interaction yielded by a two-way analysis of variance, $F(1,1482)=7.3$, $p<.01$, was plotted in Fig. 9.2. The curves, now based on the four cell means, again illustrate the greater impact of high protection on the risk-problem behavior relation than of low protection.

Replicating the cross-sectional analyses. Parallel cross-sectional hierarchical multiple regressions were carried out for the Wave-2, Wave-3, and Wave-4 data. (In Waves 3 and 4, a new, five-item measure of risk, Dropout Proneness, $\alpha=.86$, was added to the RFI, and a new, four-item measure of protection, Religiosity, $\alpha=.88$, was added to the PFI.) In each of the three subsequent data waves, the total set of predictor measures accounted for a portion of the variance in the MPBI criterion measure similar to that shown in Table 9.1 for the Wave-1 data: 25 %, 26 %, and 24 %, respectively. In each of the subsequent waves, the demographic controls were significant, but now they accounted for less than 5 % of the variance; the RFI and PFI each added a significant increment in variance accounted for; and the RFI by PFI interaction term added a further significant increment in Wave 2 and in Wave 3 (.008, $p<.001$, in each), but not in Wave 4. Thus, the four separate, cross-sectional replications yielded a similar pattern of findings in respect to both the direct and the moderator role of protective factors, except for the nonsignificant interaction in Wave 4. This robustness of outcome obtained although the sample was increasing in age from Wave 1 to Wave 4 and moving from a middle school to a high school context.

Although gender and race/ethnicity were among the demographic controls in all of these analyses, sample size was large enough to permit analyses within gender and race/ethnicity subgroups. Hierarchical multiple regressions were run for male and female students separately, and for White, Hispanic, and Black youths separately, again using the Wave-1 (1989) data. The findings for these subgroups were, with some exceptions, similar to the findings already reported for the total sample.

For female students, the total set of predictors accounted for 29 % of the variance in problem behavior involvement; for male students, it was 20 %. For both genders, the cohort measure had a significant unstandardized regression coefficient among the demographic controls. For both genders, the RFI and the PFI each added a significant increment to the R^2. And the addition of the RFI by PFI interaction term added a further significant increment (.005, $p<.05$) for the young women, but it did not reach significance for the young men.

When the analyses were carried out for the three race/ethnicity subgroups, the total set of predictors yielded R^2s of .23, .26, and .18 for Whites, Hispanics, and Blacks, respectively (all significant at $p<.001$). Among the demographic controls, cohort had a significant B coefficient for all three subgroups. The addition of the RFI and the PFI each yielded significant increments in R^2 in all groups. And the addition of the RFI by PFI interaction term yielded a further significant increment in R^2 for the Whites (.005, $p<.05$), a near significant increment for Hispanics (.005, $p<.06$), and a nonsignificant increment for Blacks. Overall, the five subgroup replications mimic those shown in Table 9.1 for the total sample, but the absence of a significant RFI by PFI interaction for male students and for Blacks is an important exception.

Analyzing the components of the MPBI. Although our primary concern in this article is with the higher order construct of problem behavior, measured here by the MPBI, the generality of the present findings can be explored by examining each of the four problem behavior components of the MPBI as a separate criterion measure. Hierarchical regressions were again carried out, but now separately for problem drinking, marijuana involvement, delinquent-type behavior, and sexual intercourse experience, again using the Wave-1 data. The pattern of findings for each behavior is consonant with that for the MPBI composite index overall: the demographic controls account for between 4 % and 12 % of the variance in the four problem behavior measures; the RFI and PFI each add a significant increment in variance accounted for (except for the PFI for sexual intercourse experience); and the RFI by PFI interaction term adds a further significant increment in variance accounted for when problem drinking (.003, $p<.05$), marijuana involvement (.004, $p<.01$), and delinquent-type behavior (.005, $p<.01$) are the criterion measures, but not when the criterion measure is sexual intercourse experience. (The sexual intercourse experience measure has the limitation of being a simple dichotomy in these analyses. It should also be mentioned that when the PFI is "unpacked," as in analyses reported later, protection does add a significant increment in variance for this measure.) The total set of predictors yielded R^2s of .16, .21, .21, and .12, respectively, for those four component behaviors, somewhat less than for the composite MPBI, but each a significant R^2 in magnitude.

Thus far, the analyses have shown that counting the number of protective factors yields a measure—the PFI—that is inversely related to adolescent involvement in problem behavior, a finding that is relatively robust over four waves of data, across gender and racial/ethnic subgroups, and across different specific problem behaviors, except for sexual intercourse experience. In addition, the role of protection as moderator of the relation of risk to problem behavior has also received support from the significant RFI by PFI interaction in the total sample analysis and in three out of the five subgroup analyses. Although small, the significant interaction effect is of substantial theoretical importance. We return to the difficulty of detecting interaction effects in field studies, and the usually small magnitudes that are found, in the Discussion.

Analyzing risk and protective factors as continuous measures. The use of cumulative indexes for risk and protection, that is, counting the number of different risk factors or protective factors, results in treating those factors as equally weighted and, in a sense, as mutually substitutable. Although useful for conceptual purposes, such analyses do obscure the differential importance that particular risk or protective factors may have in regard to adolescent problem behavior outcomes. To permit an exploration of the differential contribution of the separate measures of risk factors and protective factors, we "unpacked" the Wave-1 RFI and PFI in a series of hierarchical multiple regressions with the MPBI as the criterion. The data are shown in Table 9.2.

Table 9.2 presents the bivariate relations between each predictor measure and the criterion, the standardized beta coefficients at the final step, and the R^2 and R^2 change at each step. It is worth pointing out immediately that using the total set of 5 controls plus, now, 13 separate risk and protection measures yields a final R^2 of .48, twice the amount of variance accounted for by the 5 controls plus only the 2 RFI and PFI measures in Table 9.1. The final R^2 in Table 9.2 is similar to the level of variance in problem behavior accounted for in much of our earlier work (Jessor et al., 1991; Jessor & Jessor, 1977) using a set of about 16 predictor measures from Problem Behavior Theory. Also apparent in Table 9.2, both unpacked sets of risk factors and protective factors add a significant increment in the R^2 beyond that of the demographic controls.

At the bivariate level, there is a small negative correlation between SES and involvement in problem behavior, and a small positive correlation between cohort (grade in school or, for the most part, chronological age) and involvement in problem behavior among the demographic measures. Among the risk factors, the strongest bivariate relationship is between the criterion and Friends Models for Problem Behavior, followed by Grade Point Average and Expectations for Success. Among the protective factor measures, the most substantial predictor is Attitudinal Intolerance of Deviance, followed by Positive Orientation to School, Perceived Regulatory Controls, and Friends Models for Conventional Behavior.

The standardized betas in Table 9.2 mirror the strength of the bivariate relations. Among the demographic controls, the beta for cohort is significant; among the risk factors, Friends Models for Problem Behavior has the largest beta coefficient, with Expectations for Success, Self-Esteem, and Grade Point Average significant but considerably smaller; and, among the protective factor measures, Attitudinal Intolerance of Deviance has the largest beta, with Positive Orientation to School also being significant.

Table 9.2 Cross-sectional hierarchical multiple regression analysis of the Separate Risk Factor and Protective Factor measures with the Multiple Problem Behavior Index: Wave 1 (1989)

Step/predictor measures	Pearson r^a	β at final step[b]	R^2	R^2 change
1. Demographic Controls			.10***	
Gender	−.07	−.01		
White or Minority	−.13	.01		
Hispanic or Black	.14	.03		
Socioeconomic Status	−.17	−.02		
Cohort	.23	.05**		
2. Add Risk Factors			.43***	.328***
Expectations for Success	−.28	−.07**		
Self-Esteem	−.16	.07**		
Hopelessness	.11	.01		
Friends Models, Problem Behavior	.62	.46***		
Friend Orientation	.19	.01		
Grade Point Average	−.32	−.06**		
3. Add Protective Factors			.48***	.054***
Positive Orientation, School	−.32	−.06*		
Positive Orientation, Health	−.19	.03		
Intolerance of Deviance	−.48	−.26***		
Positive Relations, Adults	−.18	.00		
Perceived Regulatory Controls	−.24	.01		
Friends Models, Conventional Behavior	−.21	−.02		
Prosocial Activities	−.14	.00		

[a]All Pearson correlations are significant at $p \leq .01$ or better
[b] Beta values are standardized partial regression coefficients
*$p \leq .05$. ** $p \leq .01$. ***$p \leq .001$

When unpacked multiple regression analyses were run for each of the four adolescent problem behaviors separately, the pattern of findings is quite similar with regard to the relative importance of the different risk and protective factor measures. For all four problem behaviors, the risk factor measure with the consistently largest significant beta weight is Friends Models for Problem Behavior, and the protective factor measure playing that same role is Attitudinal Intolerance of Deviance. Expectations for Success has a significant beta for three of the problem behaviors, Self-Esteem for two, Hopelessness for two, and Grade Point Average for one, among the other risk factors. Among the other protective factor measures, both Positive Orientation to School and Friends Models for Conventional Behavior have significant betas for two of the problem behaviors, and Prosocial Activities has a significant beta for one of the behaviors.

At the level of the individual risk and protective factors measures, then, there is a robustness of findings, both across the composite index of problem behavior involvement and across its components, with respect to the key influence of Friends Models for Problem Behavior and Attitudinal Intolerance of Deviance, and some consistency for several of the other measures in each domain.

Longitudinal Analyses of Protection and Change in Problem Behavior

The four-wave, longitudinal design of the study provides an opportunity to examine whether antecedent protection has implications for change in adolescent involvement in problem behavior with subsequent development. Hierarchical multiple regression analysis was again used, only now with the Wave-1 MPBI score entered at Step 1 as a control, so that the criterion measure was change in the level of involvement in problem behavior in subsequent years, that is, by Wave 2, Wave 3 and Wave 4.[4] The data predicting change in MPBI by Wave 2 (1990), Wave 3 (1991), and Wave 4 (1992) are shown in Table 9.3. Because the RFI by PFI interaction term was not significant as a predictor in any subsequent year, that step is omitted from the table.

The total amount of variance explained in change in multiple problem behavior involvement declines as the time interval lengthens, from 46 % by Wave 2, to 34 % by Wave 3, to 28 % by Wave 4. As can be seen in Table 9.3, the Wave-1 MPBI score entered at Step 1 accounts for a substantial amount of variance in the subsequent MPBI scores at Waves, 2, 3, and 4. With respect to change in multiple problem behavior involvement, cohort has a significant beta coefficient in Waves 2 and 4, gender in Waves 3 and 4, and SES in Wave 4 only, when demographic controls are entered at Step 2. When the Wave-1 RFI is entered at Step 3, there is a significant increment in R^2 for all three waves, and the same is true when the Wave-1 PFI is added at Step 4. What is of special interest to note in Table 9.3 is that the PFI shows a significant beta coefficient in each of the three time intervals, whereas that is not true for the RFI in any of the time intervals.[5]

Despite stability in the MPBI score over time and development, change in multiple problem behavior involvement does, indeed, show predictability during adolescence. Of the two key theoretical measures, the RFI and the PFI, it is the antecedent number of protective factors that emerges consistently as the significant predictor of change in problem behavior involvement—the greater the earlier protection, the greater the reduction in MPBI in subsequent years.

---

[4] The Wave-2, -3, and -4 MPBI measures were constructed similarly to the Wave-1 (1989) MPBI. In each wave, there were eight outlier scores recoded to approximately three standard deviations above the mean. Alpha reliability is .74, .74, and .73 for the Wave-2, -3, and -4 MPBI, respectively. The Pearson correlation of the Wave-1 MPBI with the Wave-2, -3, and -4 MPBI is .67, .57, and .50, respectively.

[5] These analyses were replicated with a three-item MPBI, dropping the sexual experience item because it permits change in only one direction. The outcome for all three follow-up waves is essentially identical to the findings for the four-item MPBI used here.

Table 9.3 Longitudinal hierarchical multiple regression analysis of the Wave-1 (1989) Risk Factor and Protective Factor Indexes with change in Multiple Problem Behavior by Wave 2(1990), Wave 3 (1991), and Wave 4 (1992)

	Wave 2 (1990)			Wave 3 (1991)			Wave 4 (1992)		
Step/Predictor Measures	β at final step[a]	R^2	R^2 change	β at final step[a]	R^2	R^2 change	β at final step[a]	R^2	R^2 change
1. Wave-1 MPBI Score		.45***			.32***			.25***	
2. Add Demographic Controls		.46***	.005*		.33**	.006*		.27***	.016***
Gender	−.01			−.04*			−.08***		
White or Minority	.03			.03			.01		
Hispanic or Black	.02			.04			.02		
Socioeconomic Status	−.02			.00			.06*		
Cohort	−.04*			−.02			−.08***		
3. Add Wave-1 Risk Factor Index	.04	.46***	.003**	.03	.33***	.003*	.04	.27***	.004**
4. Add Wave-1 Protective Factor Index	−.07**	.46***	.003**	−.08***	.34***	.005***	−.10***	.28***	.007***

Note: MPBI=Multiple Problem Behavior Index
[a]Standardized regression coefficients, betas, are reported
*$p \leq .05$. **$p \leq .01$. *** $p \leq .001$

Discussion

Psychosocial protective factors appear to play an important role in the etiology and the developmental course of adolescent problem behavior. The present findings argue, therefore, that scientific attention should be broadened beyond its traditional preoccupation with risk factors to encompass variation in protection as well. Protective factors have been shown to relate both directly and indirectly to adolescent involvement in problem behavior—the greater the protection, the less the problem behavior—and, in interaction with risk factors, protective factors can moderate their relation to problem behavior. The overall findings show robustness across four separate waves of data, across gender and race/ethnicity subgroups, and in relation to multiple outcome criteria. The findings also obtain whether an index of the number of risk and protective factors was used or whether the actual continuous measures themselves were used.

The relation of protection to developmental change in adolescence has special significance, given the importance of problem behavior as a characteristic of that life stage. When change in involvement in problem behavior was the criterion—whether over a 1-, 2-, or 3-year interval—it was the PFI that had a significant beta weight at the final step in the regression analysis, not the RFI. What this suggests is that, although risk does have a stronger relation to variation in problem behavior involvement than protection, antecedent protection has a stronger relation to change (here diminution) in problem behavior than antecedent risk. To the extent this is true, it would have significant implications for intervention efforts seeking to reduce problem behavior involvement during adolescence.

Although not statistically significant in every analysis, the empirical support for a moderator role for protection—a significant RFI by PFI interaction—was nevertheless substantial; this may well be the most important finding of the study for theory. It corroborates a differential or variable impact of protection on the relation between risk and problem behavior—its major impact being evident when protection is high, and its influence being more limited when protection is low or absent—a pattern in accord with Rutter's (1987) earlier conceptualization.

The importance we placed on having established a significant Risk by Protection interaction may seem questionable given the small amount of additional or unique variance (about 1 %) that is accounted for in most of the analyses. As McClelland and Judd (1993) pointed out, however, "moderator effects are notoriously difficult to detect in nonexperimental field studies" (p. 377) in contrast to the apparent ease with which such effects are found in experiments. A study by Grossman et al. (1992) provides an illustration; they were able to describe "the power of... protective factors as independent predictors . . . after risk was taken into account" (p. 546) but then found it necessary to report their "second general finding. . .the absence of any interactions" (p. 547). When interactions are detected in nonexperimental studies, it is the usual case, as in the present study, that they involve only 1 % to 3 % of the total variance (Chaplin, 1991).

In a telling statistical analysis, and using the present data set as a case study, McClelland and Judd (1993) demonstrated that "jointly extreme observations are crucial for detecting interactions" (p. 382); this is precisely what is achieved by the deliberate assignment of cases in an experiment, but in field studies, the investigator has to work with whatever joint distribution of predictors happens to obtain. Given their argument, the detection of significant interactions in the present study is, indeed, noteworthy. Despite the small magnitude of those interactions, they provide strong support for the theoretical inference sought about the relation between protection and risk, namely, that protection can moderate the influence of risk on problem behavior in adolescence.

In establishing the measures of risk and protection, we followed a strategy that relied on counting the number of different risk factors or protective factors present, emphasizing thereby the amount of risk or protection rather than particular factors or particular patterns of factors. That strategy was clearly useful in revealing both the direct and moderator effects of protection and, to that extent, showing that magnitude of risk and protection is an important parameter, as others have also shown (Bry, 1983; Sameroff et al., 1987; Small & Luster, 1994). When the RFI and the PFI were unpacked (see Table 9.2), however, the differential importance of the different risk and protective factors became apparent. Although shared variance affected which measure might achieve a significant beta at the expense of another, it was clear that the most powerful protective factor was a personal control, Attitudinal Intolerance of Deviance, and next was a personal orientation and commitment to a conventional institution, Positive Orientation to School. Among the risk factors, the most powerful one was a measure of instigation in the perceived social environment, Friends Models for Problem Behavior, followed by Low Expectations for Success in regard to conventional goals, and personal vulnerability in terms of Low Self-Esteem and Hopelessness. With respect to both prevention and intervention, these findings suggest targets for program design and practices of family management.

An inquiry that engages both risk and protective factors cannot escape questioning about their separateness as domains of independent variables. The most frequent challenge is that risk and protection are really opposite ends of the same variables, hence highly correlated inversely, rather than being orthogonal. We have dealt with this problem in the introduction by specifying conceptual properties of protective factors that are deliberately different from the conceptual properties of risk factors in relation to problem behavior. Protective factors were conceptualized as variables that reflect involvement with and commitment to conventional society, that control against nonnormative activities, and that refer to activities incompatible with normative transgression. With respect to the actual measures we used to operationalize risk and protection, they seem to us to be rather clear indicators, although one or two may well be arguable. In the end, it is the empirical findings that buttress the case we have tried to make. First, the RFI and PFI share only a modest proportion (18 %) of common variance. Second, measures that might most clearly seem opposite ends of a single variable, for example, Friends Models for Problem Behavior and Friends Models for Conventional Behavior, are only correlated −.20, and indeed, in the hierarchical multiple regressions for Delinquent-Type Behavior and also for Marijuana Involvement, both of these two predictor measures retained a significant beta weight at the final step. Thus, it is neither obvious nor useful to assume that being high on one of the measures implies being low on the other.

Third, to pursue this example further, these two measures have quite different correlations with other measures, for example, with Prosocial Activities (.32 for Friends Models for Conventional Behavior and −.11 for Friends Models for Problem Behavior) or with the MPBI itself (−.21 for Friends Models for Conventional Behavior and .62 for Friends Models for Problem Behavior).

Another seemingly obvious example might be the risk factor, Grade Point Average, and the protective factor, Positive Orientation to School. Although related as expected, their correlation is, again, small (.28), and their relations to other measures are quite different. Grade Point Average correlated .36 with SES; by contrast, Positive Orientation to School correlated only .13 with SES. The respective correlations of Grade Point Average and Positive Orientation to School with Positive Orientation to Health are .14 and .42, with Attitudinal Intolerance of Deviance are .21 and .45, with Positive Relations With Adults are .10 and .30, and with Perceived Regulatory Controls are .14 and .37. The results of the present study seem to us to provide support for the heuristic value of making a conceptual distinction between protection and risk, and for efforts to operationalize that distinction with distinctive measures.

The generality of the findings for the direct effects of protection across both genders and all three racial/ethnic subgroups was pervasive. With respect to the moderator effects of protection, generality was more limited; although evident for the total sample and for the female, White, and Hispanic subgroups, a significant interaction was not found for male students or for Blacks. With respect to gender differences, a somewhat greater proportion of total variance in problem behavior is accounted for among the women than among the men (29 % vs. 20 %), but no other consistent difference was apparent. With respect to the racial/ethnic differences, the Black sample data accounted for the smallest proportion of variance of any subgroup (18 %), and the Black sample was by far the smallest subgroup ($n = 346$). But it is not obvious why no significant interaction was achieved because there was a direct effect of protection for Blacks, and Blacks also had the highest mean score on the PFI of all three ethnic groups.

The findings we have reported are limited in important ways. The less-than-desirable initial sample participation rate and the subsequent attrition certainly impose limits on the generality of the inferences that can be drawn. The conceptual effort to distinguish risk and protective factors, while salutary, could benefit from further theoretical elaboration, and the empirical support for the distinction, presented earlier, is not immune from alternative interpretation. It is also the case that the measures used, even those about the social environment, are all limited to self-reports from questionnaires, that is, all are provided by the same individual. The possibility, therefore, that common method variance has influenced the findings cannot be ruled out. It would be desirable in future research to have external validity established for the measures used. Measures independent of self-report, especially those for the ecological variables, would clearly be a step forward. Furthermore, the measurement of protection could certainly be made more exhaustive in regard to family, neighborhood, and institutional factors. Finally, deliberate sampling to maximize jointly extreme scores on the risk and protection predictors would permit stronger tests of their interaction.

Despite these limitations, the study has illuminated the role of protective factors in adolescent problem behavior and development. Greater recognition of the direct and moderator effects of protection should provide a strong stimulus for more sophisticated theorizing and, equally important, for the development of prevention and intervention efforts targeted at enhancing protection as well as at reducing risk.

Acknowledgments This study is a report from the research project supported by Grant 91-1194-88 from the William T. Grant Foundation, R. Jessor, principal investigator. Support from the MacArthur Foundation Research Network on Successful Adolescent Development Among Youth in High-Risk Settings is gratefully acknowledged. We are grateful to the officials of the school district involved for their gracious and extended cooperation. The contributions of John Donovan to this report are appreciated. The article has benefited particularly from the comments and suggestions of Gary H. McClelland and Arnold J. Sameroff.

References

Aiken, L. S., & West, S. G. (1991). *Multiple regression: Testing and interpreting interactions*. Newbury Park, CA: Sage.

Baron, R., & Kenny, D. A. (1986). The moderator-mediator variable distinction in social psychological research: Conceptual, strategic, and statistical considerations. *Journal of Personality and Social Psychology, 51*, 1173–1182.

Brook, J. S., Whiteman, M., Cohen, P., & Tanaka, J. S. (1992). Childhood precursors of adolescent drug use: A longitudinal analysis. *Genetic, Social, and General Psychology Monographs, 118*, 195–213.

Bry, B. H. (1983). Predicting drug abuse: Review and reformulation. *International Journal of the Addictions, 18*, 223–233.

Chaplin, W. F. (1991). The next generation of moderator research in personality psychology. *Journal of Personality, 59*, 143–178.

Cohen, J. (1978). Partialed products are interactions: Partialed powers are curve components. *Psychological Bulletin, 85*, 858–866.

Cohen, J., & Cohen, P. (1983). *Applied multiple regression/correlation analysis for the behavioral sciences* (2nd ed.). Hillsdale, NJ: Erlbaum.

Felix-Ortiz, M., & Newcomb, M. D. (1992). Risk and protective factors for drug use among Latino and White adolescents. *Hispanic Journal of Behavioral Sciences, 14*, 291–309.

Garmezy, N. (1985). Stress-resistant children: The search for protective factors. In J. E. Stevenson (Ed.), *Recent research in developmental psychopathology. Journal of Child Psychology and Psychiatry Book Supplement No. 4* (pp. 213–233). Oxford, England: Pergamon Press.

Garmezy, N., & Masten, A. S. (1986). Stress, competence, and resilience: Common frontiers for therapist and psychopathologist. *Behavior Therapy, 17*, 500–521.

Grossman, F. K., Beinashowitz, J., Anderson, L., Sakurai, M., Finnin, L., & Flaherty, M. (1992). Risk and resilience in young adolescents. *Journal of Youth and Adolescence, 21*, 529–550.

Hawkins, J. D., Catalano, R. F., & Miller, J. Y. (1992). Risk and protective factors for alcohol and other drug problems in adolescence and early adulthood: Implications for substance abuse prevention. *Psychological Bulletin, 112*, 64–105.

Jessor, R. (1991). Risk behavior in adolescence: A psychosocial framework for understanding and action. *Journal of Adolescent Health, 12*, 597–605.

Jessor, R. (1993). Successful adolescent development among youth in high-risk settings. *American Psychologist, 48*, 117–126.

Jessor, R., Donovan, J. E., & Costa, F. M. (1991). *Beyond adolescence: Problem behavior and young adult development*. Cambridge, England: Cambridge University Press.
Jessor, R., Graves, T. D., Hanson, R. C., & Jessor, S. L. (1968). *Society, personality and deviant behavior: A study of a tri-ethnic community*. New York: Holt, Rinehart, & Winston.
Jessor, R., & Jessor, S. L. (1977). *Problem behavior and psychosocial development: A longitudinal study of youth*. New York: Academic Press.
Luthar, S. S., & Zigler, E. (1991). Vulnerability and competence: A review of research on resilience in childhood. *American Journal of Orthopsychiatry, 61*, 6–22.
McClelland, G. H., & Judd, C. M. (1993). Statistical difficulties of detecting interactions and moderator effects. *Psychological Bulletin, 114*, 376–390.
Newcomb, M. E., Maddahian, E., & Bentler, P. A. (1986). Risk for drug use among adolescents: Concurrent and longitudinal analyses. *American Journal of Public Health, 76*, 525–531.
Pellegrini, D. S. (1990). Psychosocial risk and protective factors in childhood. *Journal of Developmental and Behavioral Pediatrics, 11*, 201–209.
Rutter, M. (1979). Protective factors in children's response to stress and disadvantage. In W. M. Kent & J. E. Rolf (Eds.), *Primary prevention of psychopathology* (Vol. 3, pp. 49–74). Hanover, NH: University Press of New England.
Rutter, M. (1987). Psychosocial resilience and protective mechanisms. *American Journal of Orthopsychiatry, 57*, 316–331.
Sameroff, A. J., Seifer, R., Baldwin, A., & Baldwin, C. (1993). Stability of intelligence from preschool to adolescence: The influence of social and family risk factors. *Child Development, 64*, 80–97.
Sameroff, A. J., Seifer, R., Barocas, R., Zax, M., & Greenspan, S. (1987). Intelligence quotient scores of 4-year-old children: Social-environmental risk factors. *Pediatrics, 79*, 343–350.
Saunders, D. R. (1956). Moderator variables in prediction. *Educational and Psychological Measurement, 16*, 209–222.
Small, S. A., & Luster, T. (1994). Adolescent sexual activity: An ecological risk-factor approach. *Journal of Marriage and the Family, 56*, 181–192.
Stacy, A. W., Newcomb, M. D., & Bentler, P. M. (1992). Interactive and higher-order effects of social influences on drug use. *Journal of Health and Social Behavior, 33*, 226–241.
Stacy, A. W., Sussman, S., Dent, C. W., Burton, D., & Flay, B. (1992). Moderators of peer social influence in adolescent smoking. *Personality and Social Psychology Bulletin, 18*, 163–172.
Werner, E. E. (1989a). Children of the garden island. *Scientific American, 260*, 106–111.
Werner, E. E. (1989b). High-risk children in young adulthood: A longitudinal study from birth to 32 years. *American Journal of Orthopsychiatry, 59*, 72–81.
Wills, T. A., Vaccaro, D., & McNamara, G. (1992). The role of life events, family support, and competence in adolescent substance use: A test of vulnerability and protective factors. *American Journal of Community Psychology, 20*, 349–374.

Chapter 10
The Cross-National Generality of Problem Behavior Theory

Richard Jessor, Mark S. Turbin, Frances M. Costa, Qi Dong, Hongchuan Zhang, and Changhai Wang

Although recent trends in studies of adolescent behavior and development reflect a "remarkable invigoration of theoretical and empirical work" (Jessor, 1998, p. 1), most of this work has been confined to Western, especially North American, populations (Alsaker & Flammer, 1999). A key challenge for the scientific study of adolescence is to extend research to non-Western societies and to undertake systematic, comparative, cross-national inquiries that can capture what is general as well as what is local and idiosyncratic in adolescent behavior and development and in their determinants.

In this article we examine the generality of an explanatory model of adolescent problem behavior in a cross-national study of adolescents from two different societies: the People's Republic of China and the United States. The model, developed in the United States, describes the relations of psychosocial protective factors and risk factors to involvement in problem behaviors such as delinquency, tobacco use, alcohol abuse, marijuana and other illicit drug use, and early sexual intercourse experience. Based on a theoretically derived conceptualization that incorporates both

---

Reprinted with permission from:
Jessor, R., Turbin, M. S., Costa, F. M., Dong, Q., Zhang, H., & Wang, C. (2003). Adolescent problem behavior in China and the United States: A cross-national study of psychosocial protective factors. *Journal of Research on Adolescence, 13*(3), 329–360.

R. Jessor (✉)
Institute of Behavioral Science, University of Colorado at Boulder, Boulder, CO, USA
e-mail: jessor@Colorado.edu

M.S. Turbin
Kalispell, MT, USA

F.M. Costa
University of Colorado Boulder, Boulder, CO, USA

Q. Dong • H. Zhang • C. Wang
Beijing Normal University, Beijing, China

R. Jessor, *The Origins and Development of Problem Behavior Theory*,
Advancing Responsible Adolescent Development,
DOI 10.1007/978-3-319-40886-6_10

contextual and individual differences in protection and risk, the model takes into account both the direct effects of protective and risk factors and the moderating influence that protection may have on the impact of exposure to risk.

The delineation of protective and risk factors in the present study emerges from a reformulation and extension of Problem Behavior Theory (Jessor, Donovan, & Costa, 1991; Jessor, Graves, Hanson, & Jessor, 1968; Jessor & Jessor, 1977). The protection-risk conceptual framework employed in the present study encompasses a more exhaustive range of protection and risk variables by including not only measures of individual-level protection and risk (e.g., attitudes, values, and beliefs) but also measures of protection and risk in the multiple social contexts that are salient in the ecology of daily adolescent life: family, peers, school, and neighborhood.

Conceptually, protective factors decrease the likelihood of engaging in problem behaviors by providing models for positive or prosocial behavior, personal or social controls against problem behavior, and an environment of support. Risk factors, in contrast, increase the likelihood of engaging in problem behavior by providing models for problem behavior, greater opportunity for engaging in problem behavior, and greater personal vulnerability to problem behavior involvement (Costa, Jessor, & Turbin, 1999; Jessor, Turbin, & Costa, 1998a, 1998b; Jessor, Van Den Bos, Vanderryn, Costa, & Turbin, 1995). Psychosocial risk and protective factors have been shown to account for substantial amounts of variance in adolescent problem behavior, and the linkages of risk and protection to problem behavior are robust in relation to multiple outcome criteria (e.g., delinquent-type behavior, problem drinking, marijuana use) for both males and females, for younger and older adolescents, across groups varying in socioeconomic status, and across race and ethnicity subgroups (White, Hispanic, and African American youth; Costa et al., 1999; Jessor et al., 1998a, 1998b; Jessor et al., 1995).

Protective factors can play an additional—indirect—role in the occurrence of adolescent problem behavior by moderating or buffering the impact of risk factors, and indeed, there is considerable empirical evidence of such moderation (Costa et al., 1999; Jessor et al., 1998a, 1998b; Jessor et al., 1995). When protection is low, the higher the risk the greater the involvement in problem behavior, but when protection is high, that relation is attenuated. The detection of such moderator or interaction effects is not only of theoretical importance but also has significant implications for intervention and policy: The strengthening of protection would assume importance along with the reducing of risk as prevention and intervention strategies for adolescent problem behavior.

The protection-risk model used in the present research is an effort to systematize work in this field. It consists of three types of protection and three types of risk that together, and in interaction, can account for variation in problem behavior. The model, and the protection and risk constructs it includes, has emerged from the series of studies on Problem Behavior Theory cited previously as well as from the recent developmental literature (e.g., Barber & Olsen, 1997). Models protection includes measures of models such as parental involvement in community groups and volunteer work, and peer models for health-enhancing behaviors such as engagement in regular exercise; controls protection includes individual-level measures of control such as attitudinal intolerance of deviance, and social environmen-

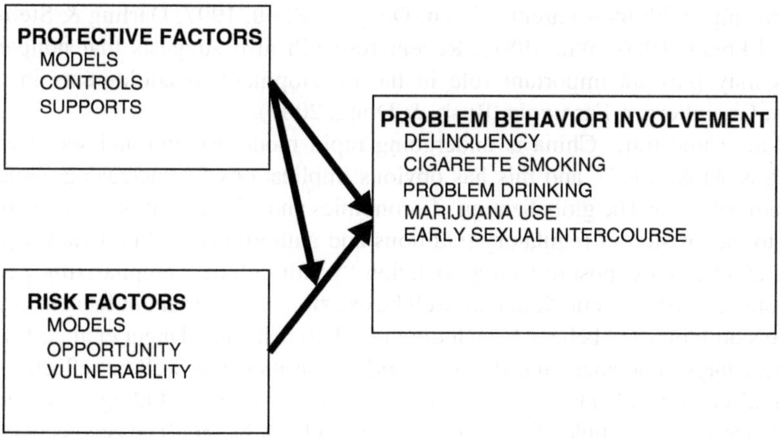

Fig. 10.1 Explanatory model of direct effects of protective factors and risk factors on adolescent problem behavior, and moderation of Risk × Protection

tal measures of controls such as predictable parental sanctions; and support protection includes measures of contextual supports such as family closeness and teacher interest in students. With regard to risk, models risk includes measures of models such as parental smoking, and peer models for alcohol use; opportunity risk includes opportunity measures such as availability of alcohol in the home and presence of gang activity in the neighborhood; and vulnerability risk includes measures of personal vulnerability such as felt stress and low self-esteem. Similar protective and risk factors have been employed in several other investigations of adolescent risk behavior (Felix-Ortiz & Newcomb, 1992; Hawkins, Catalano, & Miller, 1992; Resnick et al., 1997; Stacy, Newcomb, & Bentler, 1992; Wills, Vaccaro, & McNamara, 1992). The explanatory model, showing the direct effects of protective and risk factors on problem behavior involvement and the moderator effect of protection on the impact of risk, can be seen in Fig. 10.1.

As a site for comparative research, the People's Republic of China, the world's most populous nation, is a society that contrasts markedly with the United States in its social, political, and economic systems, as well as in the proximal social contexts in which adolescents are embedded. In China, for example, adolescents spend a major portion of their waking time in school, and schools are viewed as a context that facilitates adolescents' socioemotional development as well as cognitive and career development (Dong & Chen, 2001). Schools in China seek to maintain consistent values, standards, and requirements for adolescents' behavior and development. Schools are also enrolled as branches in national organizations such as the Young Pioneer Party and Communism Youth League that aim to inculcate prosocial values and morality education and to reinforce the schools in exercising social guidance and control over students' behavior. The structure of the family also differs across the two countries, with the prevalence of one-child families and an extremely low divorce rate in China, as against the substantial prevalence of nonintact families in the United States. Adolescents in China spend more time and have closer relationships with their parents (Chen, Dong, & Zhou, 1997; Darling & Steinberg, 1993; Ekblad, 1986; Wu, 1981). Recent research also suggests that nonparental adults may play an important role in the development of adolescents in China (Chen, Greenberger, Farruggia, Bush, & Dong, 2003).

At the same time, China is undergoing rapid modernization and social change (Wong & Mok, 1995), and this has obvious implications for increasing adolescent problem behavior. The globalization of economies and of information may be contributing to the erosion of regulatory traditions and authoritative cultural values (Unger et al., 2002), and exposure to a globalizing "youth culture," emphasizing personal autonomy and peer orientation, may well be exerting an important influence on young people's outlooks and behavior, including problem behavior (Unger et al., 2001).

These larger intersocietal differences and similarities may well be reflected in the proximal ecology of adolescent life in the two countries, including differences in prevalence and magnitude of protective factors and risk factors. The perspective of the present study is that cross-national variation in risk and protective factors can reflect significant aspects of intersocietal difference and can do so in a theoretically illuminating rather than merely descriptive fashion. Such a theoretically based, descriptive approach permits examination of intersocietal differences in mean scores on the various protection and risk measures, and of the differential salience of the several contexts in which they are assessed. But the major contribution of such an approach is the opportunity it provides for testing the adequacy of an explanatory model to account for variation in adolescent problem behavior in both societies despite whatever mean differences in protective and risk factors and, indeed, in prevalence levels of problem behavior may obtain. Exploring the generality of an explanatory model across diverse societies emphasizes their underlying, dynamic, or genotypic (Lewin, 1931) commonality rather than their obvious, apparent, or phenotypic differences—the latter being the more traditional approach to comparative cross-national research.

The bulk of studies on adolescent problem behaviors in China has been largely epidemiological, although some have examined relations among problem behaviors or associations of problem behavior with selected measures of individual differences or social environmental characteristics. Various psychosocial theories and approaches have been employed for description and interpretation of the relationships of those measures with problem behaviors, but to our knowledge, no study has employed an integrative, theory-based psychosocial model that includes comprehensive measures of risk and protection in the various contexts of adolescent life, as well as at the individual level.

Available data indicate a lower prevalence of various adolescent problem behaviors in China than in the United States, including delinquent-type behavior (Greenberger, Chen, Beam, Whang, & Dong, 2000), cigarette smoking (Hesketh, Ding, & Tomkins, 2001; Johnston, O'Malley, & Bachman, 2001; Li, Fang, & Stanton, 1996; Unger et al., 2001; Unger et al., 2002; Zhang, Wang, Zhao, & Vartainen, 2000), regular or excessive alcohol use (Guang-Ren, 1997; Johnston et al., 2001; Li, Fang, Stanton, Feigelman, & Dong, 1996; Zhimin et al., 2001), and marijuana use (Greenberger et al., 2000; Johnston et al., 2001; Zhimin et al., 2001). In general, Chinese girls report lower involvement in problem behaviors than do Chinese boys (Guang-Ren, 1997; Hesketh et al., 2001; Li, Fang, Stanton, et al.,

1996; Unger et al., 2001; Ye, 1997; Zhang et al., 2000; Zhimin et al., 2001). As has been demonstrated in the United States (e.g., Donovan & Jessor, 1985; Elliott, 1993; Jessor & Jessor, 1977), there are also, in China, positive and significant associations among alcohol use, cigarette smoking, and delinquent-type behavior such as truancy, theft, and fighting (Li, Fang, & Stanton, 1996; Li, Fang, Stanton, et al., 1996). Among the psychosocial factors linked with Chinese adolescents' involvement in various problem behaviors have been parental monitoring, peer disapproval of misconduct, peer models for problem behavior, parental smoking, availability of cigarettes, school attachment, and expectations for academic achievement (Chen, Greenberger, Lester, Dong, & Guo, 1998; Greenberger et al., 2000; Hesketh et al., 2001; Li, Fang, & Stanton, 1996; Unger et al., 2002; Zhang & Messner, 1996; Zhang et al., 2000). None of these studies, however, has explicitly investigated the contributions of the various constructs of protection and risk (i.e., models, controls, support, opportunity, vulnerability) to accounting for variation in problem behavior, none has employed a comprehensive network of measures of both context and individual, and none has assessed the moderating influence of protection on risk.

In summary, the explanatory framework used in the present cross-national, comparative study focuses on variation in risk and protective factors in the individual adolescent and in the daily ecology of adolescent life. Assessment of these risk and protective factors should permit both a description and an explanation of intra- and inter-societal variation in adolescent problem behavior in samples drawn from The People's Republic of China and the United States.

Four key questions are addressed in this study:

1. Are there differences between the Chinese sample and the U.S. sample on measures of problem behavior involvement and on measures of protective and risk factors that are consonant with the societal differences described earlier between Chinese and U.S. society?
2. Does the same set of individual-level and contextual protective factors and risk factors account for variation in problem behavior involvement in both the Chinese and the U.S. samples?
3. Do protective factors moderate, or buffer, the impact of risk factors on adolescent problem behavior in both the Chinese and the U.S. samples?
4. Does the same explanatory model account for problem behavior involvement across genders within each country sample?

Method

Study Design, Participants, and Procedures

Analyses presented in this article employed questionnaire survey data from a sample of adolescents in Beijing, China, and a sample in a large urban area in the Rocky Mountain region of the United States. The 36-page Adolescent Health and Development Questionnaire (AHDQ) was used to assess a broad range of behaviors, as well as protective and risk factors, in five domains: the individual (including beliefs, attitudes, and expectations) and four key social contexts of adolescent life—the family, the peer group, the school, and the neighborhood or community. The AHDQ is the most recent version of a questionnaire developed for use over the past several decades in both local and national sample studies (e.g., Jessor et al., 1995), with its content theoretically derived from the constructs in Problem Behavior Theory.

Members of the Chinese research team translated the AHDQ into Chinese and then back-translated it into English. Both the translation into Chinese and the back-translation were then reviewed in detail by a Chinese social scientist fluent in English at the University of North Carolina. His suggestions for revisions to the Chinese translation were forwarded to the Chinese team, and the Chinese-language version of the AHDQ was revised accordingly. In addition, the translation into Chinese was reviewed by a native Chinese student, also fluent in English, at the University of Colorado at Boulder; and the back-translation was reviewed by the U.S. team. On the basis of these multiple reviews, a few instances where the meaning may have been compromised in translation were communicated to the Chinese team. It is important to note that both of the Chinese-speaking reviewers found the Chinese team's translation of the AHDQ to be very well done, and the agreed-on equivalence of the two versions undergirds the validity of comparisons between the United States and China.

Participants in the study were 3335 students in Grades 7, 8, and 9: 1739 from China and 1596 from the United States. In each country, the sample was drawn from schools chosen in collaboration with the school district administration to best represent variation in the socioeconomic backgrounds of the students and, in the United States, to reflect the racial and ethnic composition of students in the district. In Beijing, schools were selected from two districts—one within the city and the other in the suburbs. In each district, schools known to vary in educational quality were selected to represent institutions described as above average, average, and below average. In each of the seven schools selected in Beijing and the nine schools selected in the United States, students were randomly sampled within grade for participation in the study.[1]

Active parental and personal consent was required. Letters describing the study to the parents and the students were distributed to the sampled students, and signed consent forms were returned to teachers. In the United States, all contact and consent materials were written in both English and Spanish. Questionnaires were filled out at school in large-group administration sessions proctored by research staff. In the United States, a bilingual version of the questionnaire was available for students who preferred to work in Spanish. Confidentiality was guaranteed and a Certificate of Confidentiality was obtained from the National Institutes of Health to safeguard further the privacy of responses. Each student received a token payment for filling out the questionnaire: $5 in the United States; $2, plus a gift to each school, in China.

[1]To address a possible problem of nonindependence of observations on the criterion measure within schools, we computed the intraclass correlation, which is negligible: .03 in the U.S. sample and .02 in the Chinese sample. Hence, the students' responses can be treated as independent observations.

Questionnaires were filled out by 98 % of the Chinese sample and by 74 % of the U.S. sample. In both countries, about half the participants are male (51 % in China, 47 % in the United States) and about one third were in Grades 7 (31 % and 30 %, respectively), 8 (34 %), and 9 (35 %). With respect to race and ethnicity, 45 % of the U.S. sample self-described as Hispanic, 30 % as African American, 19 % as White, 4 % as Asian American, and 2 % as American Indian. Nearly all (96 %) of the Chinese participants were of Han descent. Obviously, these local samples in both China and the United States cannot represent those countries as a whole. In what follows, use of the terms *China* and *United States* is elliptical for these specific samples of Chinese adolescents and U.S. adolescents.

Measurement of Protective Factors and Risk Factors

To keep the primary focus on assessing the applicability of the theoretical model and its major constructs, we constructed composite measures of the three types of protection (models, controls, supports) and the three types of risk (models, opportunity, and vulnerability). Each composite measure is the average of all the items in its component subscales, standardized in the combined sample and equally weighted with a mean of zero. The internal coherence of the composite protection and risk measures was established by a confirmatory factor analysis, for each measure, that showed all of its component subscales loading on a single factor. The exception was opportunity risk, which required two composite measures (see the following discussion). The proportion of variance accounted for by the various single factors ranged between .23 and .44.

The models protection composite includes the items in four multi-item component subscales (see Table 10.1) that assess parental and peer models for conventional behavior (e.g., "Does either of your parents go to church or religious services pretty regularly?" "How many of your friends do volunteer work in the community?"), and parental and peer models for health-enhancing behavior (e.g., "Do your parents [or the adults you live with] pay attention to eating a healthy diet themselves?" "How many of your friends make sure they get enough exercise?"). The controls protection composite is composed of the items in nine multiple-item subscales that assess personal and social regulation, including attitudinal intolerance of deviance (e.g., "How wrong do you think it is to cheat on tests or homework?"), parent sanctions (e.g., "If your parents knew that you had shoplifted something from a store, would you get in trouble for it?"), family controls (e.g., "Do your parents make sure they know who you're spending your time with?"), peer controls (e.g., "If you were going to do something people think is wrong, would your friends try to stop you?"), friends' disapproval (e.g., "How do most of your friends feel about someone your age drinking alcohol?"), school controls (e.g., "In your school, how strict are the rules about student behavior in class, in the halls, and on the school grounds?"), student disapproval (e.g., "What do most of the students at your school think about kids who damage school property?"), neighborhood controls (e.g., "If adults in your neighborhood saw kids doing something wrong or getting in

Table 10.1 Protective and risk factor composite measures, component subscales, and alpha reliabilities

	α	
Measure (Number of Items)	U. S. sample	Chinese sample
Protective Factors		
Models Protection (21)	.85	.82
Parent Models for Conventional Behavior (4)	.57	.58
Parent Models for Health Behavior (8)	.78	.77
Friends Models for Conventional Behavior (5)	.74	.69
Friends Models for Health Behavior (4)	.73	.67
Controls Protection (41)	.91	.91
Attitudinal Intolerance of Deviance (10)	.92	.93
Parent Sanctions (4)	.74	.53
Family Controls (8)	.78	.73
Peer Controls (4)	.81	.78
Friends Disapproval (2)	.56	.58
School Controls (3)	.64	.51
Student Disapproval (4)	.82	.84
Neighborhood Controls (3)	.72	.64
Neighborhood Disapproval (3)	.90	.81
Support Protection (16)	.85	.86
Family Support (7)	.86	.85
Friends Support (2)	.78	.62
Teacher Support (4)	.83	.78
Neighborhood Support (3)	.86	.85
Risk Factors		
Models Risk (14)	.76	.77
Family Models for Risk Behavior (2)	.22	.06
Peer Models for Risk Behavior (5)	.48	.48
School Models for Risk Behavior (5)	.88	.79
Neighborhood Models for Substance Use (2)	.56	.64
Opportunity Risk-Availability (3)	.54	.65
Availability of Cigarettes at Home (1)	–	–
Availability of Alcohol at Home (1)	–	–
Availability of Alcohol in the Neighborhood (1)	–	–
Opportunity Risk-Gangs (2)	.86	.80
Vulnerability Risk (22)	.87	.85
Felt Stress (3)	.74	.68
Depression (3)	.85	.78
Low Expectations for Success (9)	.88	.89
Low Self-Esteem (7)	.68	.68

Note: Example items of each subscale are presented in the text

trouble, would they tell the parents about it?"), and neighborhood disapproval (e.g., "How do you think most of the adults in your neighborhood feel about someone your age drinking alcohol?"). Support protection was measured by items about family support (e.g., "When you are having problems, can you talk them over with your parents?" "Are your parents interested in what you think and how you feel?"), friends' support (e.g., "When you have personal problems, do your friends try to understand and let you know they care?"), teacher support (e.g., "Do teachers at your school treat students with respect?"), and neighborhood support (e.g., "In your neighborhood, do people help each other out and look after each other?"). The alpha reliabilities of the three composite protective factors measures shown in Table 10.1 are good: .85, .91, and .85 (United States) and .82, .91, and .86 (China), respectively, in the order presented. The alphas of the subscales are also generally satisfactory, as can be seen in Table 10.1 as well.

The models risk composite is composed of the items in four multiple-item subscales that assess social models for a variety of risk behaviors (e.g., cigarette smoking, alcohol use, poor dietary habits) across the four social contexts of family, peers, school, and neighborhood (e.g., "Does anyone in your close family smoke cigarettes?" "How many of your friends use marijuana?" "How many of the students at your school get into fights?" "How much drinking is there among adults in your neighborhood, as far as you know?"). As noted earlier, opportunity risk was divided into two separate composite scales on the basis of the confirmatory factor analysis findings. Opportunity risk-availability is measured by three items that ask about perceived availability of cigarettes in the home, of alcohol in the home, and of alcohol in the neighborhood (e.g., "If you wanted to get some alcohol to drink, would you be able to get some at home?"). Opportunity risk-gangs is composed of two items that assess perceived gang activity in the neighborhood and neighborhood youths' involvement in gangs (e.g., "Do any of the kids in your neighborhood belong to gangs?"). Vulnerability risk includes the items from four multi-item component subscales, all of which measure personal vulnerability to risk, including felt stress (e.g., "In the past six months, how much stress or pressure have you felt at school?"), depression (e.g., "In the past six months, have you just felt really down about things?"), limited perceived chances for success in life (e.g., "What are the chances that you will have a happy family life?"), and low self-esteem (e.g., "On the whole, how satisfied are you with yourself?"). The alpha reliability of opportunity risk-availability is low: .54 (United States) and .65 (China); alpha reliabilities of the other three composite risk measures are all satisfactory, as can be seen in Table 10.1. Although the alphas for a few of the models risk subscales were too low to be deemed acceptable, those measures were nevertheless retained to maintain the theoretical comprehensiveness of protection and risk assessment across the multiple contexts.

Correlations among the three protective factor composites are about the same in the China sample (ranging from .46 to .61) as in the United States sample (ranging from .45 to .61). Correlations among the four composite risk factors are also similar between China (.04 to .32) and the United States (.13 to .35). Correlations between the three protective factor composites and the four risk factor composites range from .06 to -.51 in China, and from -.03 to -.52 in the United States, negative as expected (with that one exception). Although protection and risk measures do share as much as 25 % of variance, they are not opposite ends of the same dimension, and they relate differently to various criterion measures (Jessor et al., 1995). Overall, the correlations are of similar magnitude in the two country samples.

Measurement of Adolescent Problem Behavior Involvement

The composite Multiple Problem Behavior Index (MPBI) criterion used in this report is an average of *T*-scored (M=50, *SD*=10 in the combined sample) measures of adolescents' involvement in three different types of problem behavior: (a) delinquent behavior, including theft, vandalism, and physical aggression (alpha=.84 United States, .82 China); (b) cigarette smoking, based on respondents' reports of frequency and amount of smoking in the past month and the past year (alpha=.79 United States, .84 China); and (c) problem drinking, based on self-reports of frequency of drunkenness, frequency of high-volume drinking (four or more drinks per occasion), and negative consequences of drinking, such as getting into trouble with parents or having problems with friends or at school because of drinking (alpha=.69 United States, .64 China). Alpha reliability of this three-component MPBI is .69 in the United States and .64 in China, with an average interitem correlation of .42 (United States) and .37 (China). Sexual intercourse experience was measured in the United States but not in China. Although marijuana use was measured in both countries, almost no Chinese participants reported using the drug. These latter two component behaviors, therefore, have been omitted from the composite MPBI for these comparative analyses. Although the MPBI is the key criterion measure of adolescent problem behavior in the following analyses, analyses of each of its three components are also presented.

Analytic Procedure

The primary analytic procedure used to examine the applicability of the explanatory model to variation in adolescent problem behavior is hierarchical multiple regression, carried out on the sample data from each country. Hierarchical regression lends itself to estimating interaction or moderator effects (Cohen & Cohen, 1983). Sociodemographic measures (gender, grade in school, intact family, socioeconomic status, and school attended) were entered at the first step of the regression.[2] The theoretical predictors—the three composite protective and the four composite risk factor measures—were entered, in that order, in the next two steps to examine their association with problem behavior involvement.[3] At Step 4, cross-products of all protective and risk factors were entered to examine whether protective factors were, indeed, moderators of the effects of risk factors and to determine whether those moderator effects provided a significant additional increment in variance accounted for. At Step 5, the model was tested for gender differences by entering all cross-products of

[2] There is essentially no ethnic variation in the Chinese sample, but we examined ethnic variation in the U.S. sample and found it virtually uncorrelated with problem behavior involvement. No measure of ethnicity would have been significant in the regression analyses; therefore, it was omitted.

[3] The order of entry of the protective factors and risk factors is, of course, arbitrary in testing the explanatory model. We have chosen to enter protection before risk to draw attention to protection in contrast to the more general preoccupation with risk. By reversing the order of entry in an additional hierarchical regression, it is possible to establish the unique variance contributed by each.

gender with each of the protective and risk factors and with their interactions. After all interaction terms were tested for significance in the last two steps of the regression, the equation was reestimated, omitting the nonsignificant interactions unless they were components of significant three-way (Gender × Protection × Risk) interactions.

Results

Presentation of the results is organized in the order of the research questions posed in the introduction. First, we examine descriptive differences between the Chinese and the U.S. samples on various measures, including the theoretical predictor measures of protective and risk factors, and the criterion measures of problem behavior involvement. Next, we explore the multivariate account of problem behavior involvement provided by the theoretical measures, the protective factors, and risk factors in the two samples separately. Third, we assess whether moderating effects of protective factors on the relation of risk factors to problem behavior are evident in the data. Fourth, we examine the generality of the explanatory model across genders within each sample. Next, we "unpack" the multiple problem behavior criterion measure and analyze its components to assess how well the model applies to each problem behavior in each sample. Finally, we unpack the composite protective and risk factor measures to see whether their component subscales have differential importance across the two samples.

Differences Between the Chinese Sample and the U.S. Sample on Descriptive and Theoretical Measures

With regard to descriptive differences, the impact of China's one-child policy is evident in the finding that the median number of children in the families in the Chinese sample is 1, compared with a median of 2 in the U.S. sample. Of the Chinese students, 83 % were from families with both biological parents in the home, whereas the corresponding figure for U.S. students was only 45 %. The average level of parental education in the Chinese sample was high school completion, whereas in the U.S. sample it was at least some education beyond high school (all mean differences reported in this section are significant at $p < .001$). Most of the Chinese participants (77 %) do not attend religious services, and only 5 % reported that their parents attend services pretty regularly; in the U.S. sample, most participants (55 %) reported attending religious services at least two or three times a month, and 54 % reported that their parents attend services pretty regularly. In China, the great majority of study participants (about 75 %) reported having a father who smokes cigarettes and 6 % reported a mother who smokes; in the United States, about 25 % reported having a father who smokes and 25 % reported having a mother who smokes.

Only 27 % of the Chinese students had missed 1 or more days of school in the previous semester, compared with 80 % of the U.S. students. Chinese students reported spending twice as much time doing homework as the U.S. students. Most participants in China (57 %) study 6 hr a week or more, with 36 % reporting 8 or more hr, whereas most U.S. participants (62 %) study 3 hr a week or less, with only 8 % reporting 8 or more hr. Chinese participants reported fewer models for student-to-student harassment in school than did U.S. participants. The latter three differences are consistent with the characterization of Chinese social structure as having a greater level of social controls in the schools.

On a self-rating of general health from poor to excellent, the average response among the Chinese students was good, whereas the average response for the U.S. students was very good. Fewer of the Chinese adolescents said they had been taught about AIDS and HIV in school (57 % vs. 72 % in the United States), fewer reported knowing how to prevent AIDS and HIV (59 % vs. 78 %), and fewer indicated willingness to be in a class with a student with AIDS/HIV (18 % vs. 50 %).

At the descriptive level, then, the Chinese participants come from smaller, intact families, whose backgrounds involve less formal education, different religious traditions, and more conventional behavior, compared with U.S. adolescents. In regard to problem behavior—as indicated by their scores on the MPBI and on each of its components—Chinese students, especially girls, reported lower levels of involvement than American students. Theoretically consistent with the Chinese adolescents' lower levels of problem behavior, they also have higher means scores on protective factors and lower mean scores on two of the risk factors than the U.S. adolescents (see Table 10.2). From what has been reported about Chinese soci-

Table 10.2 Group means on protective factors, risk factors, and problem behavior measures

	U.S. sample		Chinese sample	
Measure	Boys ($n=753$)	Girls ($n=843$)	Boys ($n=883$)	Girls ($n=856$)
Protective Factors				
Models Protection	49.72[a]	49.05[a]	51.40[b]	49.71[a]
Controls Protection	45.40[a]	48.75[b]	50.95[c]	54.24[d]
Support Protection	48.51[a]	50.09[b]	50.29[b]	50.91[b]
Risk Factors				
Models Risk	50.66[ab]	51.52[a]	49.50[bc]	48.48[c]
Opportunity Risk-Availability	49.73[ab]	49.23[a]	50.65[b]	50.31[ab]
Opportunity Risk-Gangs	52.09[a]	51.99[a]	49.15[b]	47.23[c]
Vulnerability Risk	48.21[a]	48.60[a]	51.16[b]	51.74[b]
Problem Behaviors				
Multiple Problem Behavior Index	51.84[a]	51.24[a]	49.87[b]	47.27[c]
Delinquent Behavior	53.48[a]	51.16[b]	49.48[c]	46.40[d]
Smoking Involvement	50.80[a]	51.17[a]	50.38[a]	47.63[b]
Problem Drinking	51.28[a]	51.41[a]	49.60[b]	47.76[b]

Note: For consistency in comparing group means in this table, each measure is transformed to a *T* score with overall mean of 50

[a, b, c, d]Superscripts not shared by group means indicate significant differences by Scheffé multiple-range test with "experimentwise" alpha set at .05

ety—that there is more concern for conventionality and more control against normative transgression—these differences are as expected. On the other two risk factors, Chinese participants reported greater opportunity availability, reflecting the greater availability of cigarettes and alcohol in the home (use of alcohol and tobacco by adolescents is not prohibited in China, but heavy use is discouraged by parents) and greater vulnerability, reflecting lower expectations for success and lower self-esteem in the Chinese sample. With these two exceptions, the mean differences in reported levels of protection and risk are theoretically consonant with the differences in reported involvement in problem behavior between the Chinese and the U.S. samples, providing initial support for the relationships specified by the explanatory framework.

Testing the Explanatory Model of Adolescent Problem Behavior Involvement in the Chinese and U.S. Samples

To examine whether the explanatory model of problem behavior involvement applies across the two samples, we regressed the MPBI on the theoretical measures—the three protective factors and four risk factors—in a hierarchical multiple regression analysis for each sample. The final regression model, representing the influence of each variable with all other variables (including interaction terms) present in the equation, is shown in Table 10.3. The final model accounts for a substantial proportion of the variance in adolescent problem behavior involvement in both samples: 46 % in the United States and 44 % in China. Despite the use of composite measures—a conservative approach that limits the number of measures employed and weights each component item equally—nearly half the variance is accounted for.

In Table 10.3 we present both standardized regression coefficients (betas) and unstandardized regression coefficients (B-weights). This permits us to compare betas at Step 3 before the interaction terms are entered and to examine interactions, at Steps 4 and 5, that require use of unstandardized regression coefficients (Aiken & West, 1991, pp. 40–47). The bivariate correlations in Table 10.3 show that all of the composite protective factor measures have the expected negative relations with the MPBI, and that all of the composite risk factor measures have the expected positive relations with the MPBI; their absolute magnitudes range from .18 to .54, and all are significant. Thus, at the bivariate level, each protective and risk factor is associated, as expected, with problem behavior involvement in each sample.

Sociodemographic measures, entered at Step 1 of the regression analysis, accounted for 6 % of the variance in problem behavior involvement in the U.S. sample and 9 % in the Chinese sample. The three composite measures of protective factors, entered at Step 2, accounted for an additional 25 % of the variance in the U.S. sample and 17 % in the Chinese sample. The four composite measures of risk factors, entered at Step 3, accounted uniquely for another 8 % (United States) and 6 % (China) of variance beyond the variance accounted for by the already-entered protective factors and sociodemographic measures. (Because the protective and risk factors share common variance, their order of entry was reversed in additional analyses to establish

Table 10.3 Hierarchical regression of multiple problem behavior involvement on composite protective factors and risk factors in the U.S. and Chinese samples

		U.S. Sample					*Chinese Sample*				
Step		*r*	*β,[a] Step 3*	*B,[b] Final Step*	ΔR^2	R^2	*r*	*β,[a] Step 3*	*B,[b] Final Step*	ΔR^2	R^2
1	Sociodemographic background				.06	.06				.09	.09
	Gender	−.03	.01	.20			−.21***	−.13***	−.59***		
	Grade in school	.17***	.03	.65			.15***	.01	.32*		
	Intact family	−.09***	−.04	−.65			−.08***	−.03	−.76*		
	Socioeconomic status	−.04	.02	.04			−.04*	.02	.16		
	School attended[c]										
2	Protective factors[d]				.25	.31				.17	.27
	Models protection	−.24***	.09**	1.40**			−.21***	.05*	.44		
	Controls protection	−.54***	−.39***	−6.25***			−.49***	−.35***	−3.64***		
	Support protection	−.35***	.05	.73			−.32***	.04	.24		
3	Risk factors				.08	.38				.06	.32
	Models risk	.46***	.23***	3.33***			.40***	.22***	3.17***		
	Opportunity risk—availability	.29***	.05*	.59*			.18***	.01	.27		
	Opportunity risk—gangs	.29***	.11***	.69**			.18***	.07**	.50***		
	Vulnerability risk	.35***	.14***	1.83***			.29***	.15***	1.88***		
4	Protection × Risk interactions[e]				.07	.45				.09	.41
	Controls Protection × Models Risk			−4.60***					−5.88***		
	Controls Protection × Opportunity Risk–Availability			−1.77**							
	Controls Protection × Opportunity Risk–Gangs			−1.14**							
	Controls Protection × Vulnerability Risk			−3.69***					−2.81***		
5	Gender interactions[e]				.01	.46				.03	.44
	Gender × Controls Protection			1.62***					.86**		
	Gender × Support Protection			−1.50***							
	Gender × Models Risk								−.98***		
	Gender × Vulnerability Risk								−.78**		
	Gender × Controls Protection × Models Risk								1.77***		
	Gender × Controls Protection × Vulnerability Risk								1.84***		

Notes. $N = 1{,}352$ (U.S.), 1,630 (China).
[a]Standardized regression weights at Step 3, before interaction terms are entered.
[b]Unstandardized regression weights are displayed; standardized weights are deemed inappropriate with interaction terms (see Aiken & West, 1991, pp. 40–47).
[c]Dummy variables for nine schools in the United States, seven in China; only one, in China, has a significant regression weight.
[d]When protective factors are entered after risk factors—that is, when the order of entry is reversed—variance accounted for uniquely by protective factors = .08*** (United States), .07*** (China).
[e]Only significant interactions are included.
*$p \leq .05$;
**$p \leq .01$.
***$p \leq .001$. All ΔR^2 and R^2 values are significant at $p \leq .001$.

the unique variance accounted for by each. When the order of entry of protective and risk factors was reversed, protective factors accounted uniquely for 8 % of variance in the U.S. sample and 7 % in the Chinese sample, about the same as the unique influence, 8 % and 6 %, shown at Step 3 in Table 10.3 for the risk factors.)

The composite protective factor of controls protection has a significant coefficient in the final regression model in both samples. All four composite risk factors are significant in the U.S. sample, and three of the four are significant in the Chinese sample. The standardized coefficients, second column for each sample, show that controls protection is the most powerful measure and that models risk is next in both of the samples. Vulnerability risk follows in importance in both samples. In the U.S. sample only, models protection has a significant positive weight, although its bivariate correlation is negative, indicating its role as a suppressor variable, improving the overall model by subtracting irrelevant variance from the other predictors (Cohen & Cohen, 1983). The apparent importance of any particular protective or risk factor is, of course, affected by the presence or absence of other measures in the regression model. In light of the fact that the bivariate correlations of the protective and risk factors with the criterion measure are all statistically significant, it is possible that the nonsignificance of some of the partial regression weights generated by the multivariate analyses may be due to their shared variance with the other predictors.

In terms of amount of variance accounted for, and in terms of which composite protective and risk factors are most important in the account, the explanatory model appears essentially the same across the two samples.

Testing for the Moderator Effect of Protection on the Relation of Risk to Problem Behavior

The moderating effect of protective factors on the relation of risk factors to problem behavior was evaluated at Step 4 with the entry of all 12 of the Protection × Risk cross-products. When all of these interaction terms were added at Step 4, the increase in R^2 was significant at $p < .05$. The model was then recomputed, omitting the nonsignificant interaction terms. The unstandardized regression coefficients for this final model are shown in Table 10.3 in the third column for each sample. The significant interactions accounted for an additional 7 % of variance in the U.S. sample and 9 % in the Chinese sample. This is a large moderator effect for a nonexperimental field study, according to McClelland and Judd (1993), as large as the direct effect of either protection or risk. Controls protection not only has a strong direct protective effect with regard to problem behavior involvement, as shown in Step 2, but it also buffers the impact of all four of the risk factors in the U.S. sample and of two of the risk factors—models risk and vulnerability risk—in the Chinese sample, as shown in Step 4. That is, when controls protection is high, the influence of those risk factors is attenuated. These are the first data to our knowledge to show that moderator effects obtain in a Chinese sample as well, and the magnitude of these effects in both samples is impressive. These similar moderator results add further evidence for the generality of the model across the two country samples.

The moderator effect in each sample is illustrated in Fig. 10.2, which shows the interaction of controls protection with a combined risk factors score for each sample. The combined score is the mean of the risk factor measures with which controls protection has significant interactions, four measures in the United States and two in China. The distributions of controls protection and of the combined risk score were trichotomized within each sample to define groups as low, medium, and high on those measures. The figure shows the mean MPBI score for groups of participants in the lowest third of protection scores (top two lines) and the highest third of protection scores (bottom two lines) who had low, medium, or high combined risk scores, respectively. As the figure shows, the relation of risk to problem behavior involvement within each sample (United States, dashed lines; China, solid lines) is

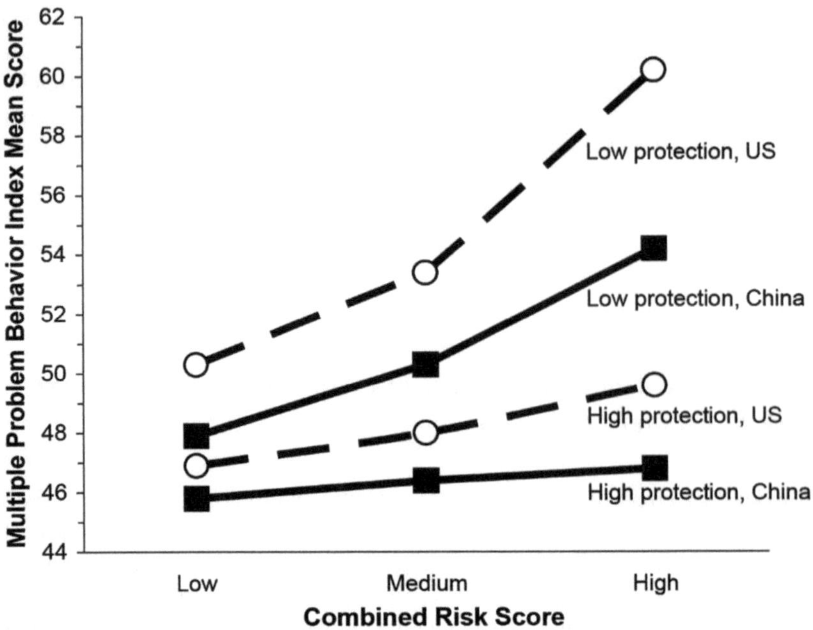

Fig. 10.2 Moderation of Combined Risk Score × Controls Protection: U.S. Sample and Chinese Sample

stronger (steeper) at low levels of protection, and it diminishes when protection is high. In other words, when protection is high, the impact of risk is attenuated. Conversely, for each sample, the difference in problem behavior involvement between low and high protection is greatest when risk is high; when risk is low, the influence of protection is less important. The figure also indicates that the lower problem behavior involvement of Chinese participants compared with U.S. participants, noted earlier, obtains at all levels of protection and risk.

Testing the Generality of the Model Across Genders

The regression models for both samples that best fit the data when boys and girls were combined are nearly the same. Because there is a substantial difference between boys and girls in mean problem behavior involvement in the Chinese sample (girls significantly lower), we tested whether the same regression model fits the data for each gender within each sample. At Step 5, we tested whether protection and risk measures had significant interactions with gender (coded -1 for boys, 1 for girls) and whether each measure was significant for both genders. All of the significant effects of protective factors, risk factors, and Protection × Risk interactions, noted in Steps 2,3, and 4, are significant for both genders in both samples.[4] Although the gender interactions shown at Step 5 in Table 10.3 indicate that six effects are stronger for one gender than for the other in at least one sample, the magnitude of all the gender interactions is small, with t values around 3.

In short, the same protective factors and most of the same risk factors are significantly associated with problem behavior involvement for both boys and girls in both samples. In both samples, also, controls protection moderates the impact of risk factors for both genders. Each set of composite theoretical predictors accounts uniquely for 6 % to 8 % of variance in each sample for both genders. The strength of the effects of the protective and risk factors differs little between genders. Overall, the model is similar across samples, and now across genders within each sample. And the overall model accounts for a substantial proportion (about 45 %) of the variance in adolescent problem behavior involvement in both samples.[5]

Unpacking the Composite Measure of Multiple Problem Behavior Involvement (MPBI)

Although the primary focus of this study is on the higher order construct of multiple problem behavior involvement, the MPBI, it is important to examine the applicability of the explanatory model to the component behaviors included in the overall index. As noted earlier, their interrelations averaged .42 (United States) and .37 (China). The regression analysis described earlier was repeated for each of the three components of the MPBI separately: delinquent behavior, cigarette smoking, and problem drinking (not tabled; tables are available from the authors). The protection-risk model accounts for 41 % of the variance in delinquent behavior in the U.S. sample and 36 % in the Chinese sample, and there are significant increments of 2 % (United States) and 3 % (China) of variance accounted for by Protection × Risk interactions. In the analysis of cigarette smoking, results are similar to the previous analyses, despite lower bivariate correlations between the predictors and the criterion (.08 to .35) and less total variance accounted for: 27 % (United States) and 23 % (China). Protection × Risk interactions are relatively strong, accounting for a

[4] To determine whether the coefficient for each gender is significantly different from zero, each significant regression weight for a gender interaction at Step 5 in Table 3 (e.g., for Gender × Controls Protection: 1.62 for the U.S. sample, .86 for the Chinese sample) was added to (for girls) or subtracted from (for boys) the tabled coefficient for the relevant predictor (for controls prediction: — 6.25 for the U.S. sample, — 3.64 for the Chinese sample) to yield the coefficient representing the effect within each gender. Dividing that coefficient by its standard error gives a t statistic for testing its significance for that gender.

[5] A broader criterion measure of multiple problem behavior involvement that includes two more components—marijuana use and sexual activity—is available in the U.S. data. In supplementary analyses of the U.S. sample data, using the broader criterion measure, the same protective and risk factors, along with their interaction effects, account for an even greater amount—51 %—of variance.

significant increment of 7 % in each sample. Finally, in the analysis of problem drinking, despite lower bivariate correlations of the theoretical predictors with this criterion (.08 to .38) than with the MPBI, results are similar, and the protection-risk model accounts for 27 % (United States) and 26 % (China) of the variance. Protection × Risk interactions account for a significant increment of 5 % (United States) and 8 % (China) of the variance in problem drinking.

In summary, results from analyses of the three component problem behaviors in the MPBI are consistent with the earlier analysis of the composite MPBI itself. The pattern of significant protective and risk factors is nearly the same, and controls protection continues to be a consistent moderator of the various risk factors for each component behavior in each country sample.

Unpacking the Composite Measures of Protection and Risk

Each composite measure of protection or risk used in the present study summarizes influences from the individual and from the different social contexts. Composite measures, although best representing the theoretical constructs, may obscure possible differences in the relative importance of the protection components or the risk components. In an auxiliary hierarchical regression analysis, we unpacked the 7 composite predictor measures shown in Table 10.1 and entered the 29 separate protective and risk factor component subscales instead. This alternative approach permits each protective or risk factor subscale to be optimally weighted in the regression equation to maximize the criterion variance accounted for, in contrast to the equal weighting that each protective or risk factor item had in its composite measure. Now the relationship between each specific protective or risk factor subscale and the MPBI criterion measure can be seen.

In these results (not tabled; tables are available from the authors), total variance accounted for in multiple problem behavior involvement is substantially increased as would be expected—to 68 % (from 46 %) in the U.S. sample and to 62 % (from 44 %) in the Chinese sample. Increases of 11 % (United States) and 7 % (China) are due to the main effects of protection and risk, and the remaining increases are accounted for by numerous Protection × Risk interactions. (Because the ratio of sample size to number of predictor variables is small, about 5 to 1, some portion of that account is probably due to capitalization on random sampling error.) With respect to protection, in both samples, the strongest predictor (based on comparison of *t* values) in this unpacked, subscale analysis is an individual-level protection measure—attitudinal intolerance of deviance, a measure of controls protection. The measure of support from teachers is the next strongest protective factor in both samples. In the Chinese sample, disapproval of problem behavior by adults in the neighborhood is a strongly significant protective factor, and family controls and friends models for conventional behavior are also significant. In the U.S. sample, family support is a significant protective factor. With respect to risk, the two most important risk factors for both samples in this unpacked analysis are friends models for risk behavior and school models for risk behavior; this is consistent with the relative strength of models risk in the main analyses. In the Chinese sample, an individual-level measure of vulnerability risk—depression—is also a strongly significant risk factor, and family models for risk behavior and neighborhood gang activity are also significant risk factors. In both samples, then, the most important component protective factors are individual-level controls and teacher support, and the most important component risk factors are models provided by friends and by peers at school.

When each of the three component behaviors of the MPBI was then analyzed with these unpacked subscale predictors, similarly high proportions of variance are accounted for in delinquent behavior (64 % in the U.S. sample, 53 % in the Chinese sample), cigarette smoking (55 % and 47 %), and problem drinking (53 % and 54 %), with many of the same protective and risk factors being significant.

Discussion

A theory-derived explanatory model of psychosocial protection and risk has been shown to provide a substantial account of variation in problem behavior involvement among adolescent samples in both the People's Republic of China and the United States. Not only was the magnitude of the account similar in both samples, but the same measures of protection and risk were related to problem behavior in the same way in both. In addition, protection was shown to serve as a moderator, or buffer, of risk in both the Chinese and the U.S. adolescent samples. Overall, the findings provide support for the generality of the explanatory model across these samples of adolescents from two very different societies.

The articulation of three types of protection—models, controls, and supports—and three types of risk—models, opportunity, and vulnerability—proved to be a useful and illuminating systematization. Assessment of those constructs, at both the individual level and in the key contexts of adolescent life, yielded theoretically relevant measures that were internally coherent, relatively independent, and significantly related to the multiple problem behavior criterion. Most important, perhaps, is that the employment of such differentiated measures in this study made it possible to determine which types of protection and which types of risk were most important in accounting for variation in adolescent problem behavior, and which types of protection moderated which types of risk. This kind of theory-based differentiation should have salutary implications for future research on risk and protective factors.

The explanatory model and its construct-relevant measures also make it possible to examine the relative importance of protection versus risk as influences or determinants of adolescent problem behavior. The data from the hierarchical regression analyses in Table 10.3 indicate that the composite measures of protection accounted for 8 % (United States) and 7 % (China) unique variance, and the composite measures of risk accounted for 8 % (United States) and 6 % (China) unique variance. In terms of their direct effects, protection and risk are essentially equivalent influences on adolescent problem behavior in these samples. It is important to note, however, that protection also has an indirect effect on adolescent problem behavior, through its moderation of the impact of risk. The moderator effect of protection, as shown at Step 4 in Table 10.3, adds an additional increment of 7 % (United States) and 9 % (China) to the explained variance. Obviously, these findings reflect the particular measures used in this study and the particular criterion involved, but they do make a compelling case for rethinking the preoccupation with risk (and risk reduction) among researchers and interventionists in this field, and for giving greater attention to protection (and promotion) in efforts to understand and influence adolescent involvement in problem behavior.

Beyond the important role played by protection in general, it is a key finding of this study that the type of protection that is most influential in regard to adolescent involvement in problem behavior has to do with the regulation of transgression, that is, what we have called controls protection. Compared with models protection and support protection, it not only has the strongest direct effect in both country samples, but when all measures are in the final regression equation, it is the only type of protection that moderates risk, indeed, all the types of risk that were measured in the U.S. sample and both models risk and vulnerability risk in the Chinese sample (see Table 10.3).

Among the significant component subscales of controls protection, when the construct was unpacked, were attitudinal intolerance of deviance at the individual level and, in the Chinese sample only, two social context subscales—family controls and neighborhood disapproval. Historically, attitudinal intolerance of deviance has been a strong and consistent individual-level predictor of adolescent problem behavior involvement (e.g., Jessor et al., 1991; Jessor & Jessor, 1977). The greater relevance of family controls to adolescent problem behavior in the Chinese sample versus the U.S. sample appears consistent with Chinese "cultural expectations of filial piety and kin obligation" (Wong, 1995, p. 53), with numerous studies showing that Chinese parents are more controlling and authoritarian compared with Western parents (Dornbusch et al., 1987; Kelley, 1992; Lin & Fu, 1990) and that parental authoritarianism may have a positive effect on social adjustment and academic achievement in Chinese children (Chen et al., 1997; Ho, 1986); also, there may be in Chinese society "strong neighborhood organizations" (Rojek, 2001, p. 89) and, more generally, a "long tradition of social organization and social control" (Rojek, 2001, p. 101).

Although support protection was not a significant predictor in the final regression equation for the main analysis of multiple problem behavior involvement, component subscales of that construct were shown to account for problem behavior involvement when the composite measure was unpacked. Among the four support protection subscales, perceived teacher support was a significant protective factor in both the Chinese and the U.S. samples, and in the United States, but not in China, perceived family support was also protective against problem behavior. The importance of "the behavior and attitudes of teachers" (Greenberger et al., 2000, p. 385) and of the role of teachers in adolescent development in China (Chen et al., 2003) is consonant with the teacher support subscale finding in the Chinese sample.

In the contemporary literature on adolescent socialization, emphasis has been placed on two protection constructs similar to those we have specified in our explanatory model: connectedness and regulation (Barber, 1997; Barber & Olsen, 1997); the former is related to our support protection construct, and the latter to our controls protection construct. With regard to controls protection, Barber and Olsen (1997) noted that "regulation experienced in the family and/or in other social contexts would be protective against externalized problem behaviors" (p. 290), a comment consistent with our own findings. What the present study adds is a demonstration of the relatively greater importance of controls protection, compared with support protection, in regulating problem behavior involvement in these adolescent samples.

In contrast to the relatively weak role of models protection as protective against problem behavior involvement, models risk emerges as the most important type of risk for involvement in problem behavior in both country samples. Peer models for risk behavior and schoolmate models for risk behavior have significant weights in the unpacked analyses of subscales, as would have been expected from the large literature on peer models as a key risk factor for adolescent problem behavior in the United States (e.g., Costa et al., 1999; Greenberger et al., 2000; Jessor et al., 1998b; Jessor et al., 1995; Kandel, 1985; Oetting & Beauvais, 1987) and among Chinese adolescents (e.g., Greenberger et al., 2000).

This effort to examine the reach of an explanatory model has engaged adolescents from a society markedly different from the United States in economic system, social organization, cultural traditions, family structure, and so on—a severe challenge to demonstrating the generality of a theoretical framework. Data from the AHDQ documented numerous mean differences between the sample of Chinese adolescents and the sample of U.S. adolescents, and many of those were described at the outset of the Results section. In addition to this eclectic approach to describing differences between the two samples, the samples were also described in the language of the theoretical framework, that is, in terms of its constructs of protective factors, risk factors, and problem behavior. That description showed in Table 10.2 that problem behavior was less prevalent in the Chinese sample than in the U.S. sample, as expected, and that, as would then be expected from the theory, protection was higher in the Chinese sample and, with some exceptions, risk was lower. This latter theory-based approach to description made clear not only that the two samples came from social contexts that differed markedly on a variety of obvious characteristics, but that the samples differed significantly in mean levels of the theoretical constructs, posing a further challenge to demonstrating generality. That the explanatory model was in many ways invariant across the two samples, despite these differences, strengthens the claim for its generality.

It is obvious, however, that the complexity of the two societies and the broad differences between them in traditional values and culture cannot be fully captured by a selected set of measures of protection and risk, nor should the emphasis on the explanatory model having generality across the samples obscure important issues that require further analysis. For example, the sociodemographic measures—gender, grade in school, and intact family—were all significant in the final regression model in the Chinese sample but not in the U.S. sample, and the increment in variance explained by the measures of protection and risk was larger in the U.S. sample (40 %) than in the Chinese sample (32 %). Such issues deserve additional attention.

The inferences that can be drawn from the findings we have presented are constrained by several of the study's limitations. First, as we pointed out in the Methods section, it is essential to emphasize that our samples were drawn from local, urban settings in each country, and they do not represent China or the United States as nations. We have tried throughout to refer to the "Chinese sample" and the "U.S. sample" to forestall unwarranted conclusions about Chinese and U.S. societies as a whole. The data are appropriate only for inferences about the samples assessed and the limited, urban, school-based populations they may represent. A further limitation inherent in all cross-national research is the possibility that, despite the care taken with the translation process, some of the measures could have different meanings for the Chinese and the U.S. adolescent respondents. This issue of the meaning equivalence of measurement across groups is a refractory one (see Knight & Hill, 1998) that resists easy resolution (and indeed is one that obtains even between any two individuals in the same group), and it cannot be ruled out entirely. Knight and Hill (1998) urged that evidence in support of equivalence be provided by comparison across groups of the reliability coefficients of measures, as well as of their validity coefficients. The similarity across the U.S. and Chinese samples of the alpha reliability coefficients, shown in Table 10.1, for both the composite and the subscale measures, and of the bivariate "validity" coefficients for the composite measures, shown in Table 10.3, is supportive in that regard. In addition, the congruent pattern of explanatory findings in both country samples, and for both genders, is a source of further reassurance about meaning equivalence.

A third limitation stems from the fact that the measures of both the predictor and criterion variables are based on self-reports, and the obtained relationships could have been influenced by common method variance. With regard to this limitation, we were able to compare participants' self-reports with independent parent reports on similar measures. Parents of a subsample of the adolescent participants ($n = 316$, United States; $n = 347$, China) completed a short questionnaire assessing protective factors and risk factors in their children's social contexts—family, school, peers, and neighborhood. Measures parallel to the measures from the child's AHDQ could be constructed for three protective factors and three risk factors. Correlations of student self-reports and the corresponding parent reports revealed a significant degree of consistency, with most of the correlations ranging between .15 and .34 in both the U.S. and Chinese samples. To that extent, they constitute some indication of external validity of the self-reports.

It is possible, also, to argue that the veridicality of the self-reports might differ between the two samples given the Chinese cultural emphasis on conformity and normative adherence and, hence, the greater social undesirability of acknowledging normative transgressions such as problem behavior. In this regard, every effort was made to assure participants about the confidentiality of their questionnaire responses and the privacy of the data. In addition, the parent substudy indicated that the parent-child correlations were similar in both China and the United States. Furthermore, it could be counterargued that the same Chinese cultural tradition of normative adherence would militate against giving deceptive responses on a questionnaire, a normative transgression in itself. Although it is not possible to rule out differential veridicality in the Chinese-U.S. samples' self-reports of problem behavior, it needs reminding that the fundamental concern of the study is with relations among variables rather than with their absolute mean levels, and in that regard the findings are compellingly similar in both samples.

With respect to the analytic method used, ordinary least squares (OLS), the substantial skewness of the problem behavior criterion measure could raise a question about whether OLS is appropriate, and especially whether its application might yield interactions that are in fact spurious. A log transformation of the criterion measure did reduce the skewness, and a further OLS analysis yielded the same interactions. Beyond this, we also undertook a tobit analysis, considered more appropriate for use with skewed outcome measures. The results of the tobit analysis continued to show significance for three of the four Protection × Risk interactions in the U.S. sample; the fourth had a significance level of $p = .06$. In the Chinese sample, one of the two significant Protection × Risk interactions retained significance in the tobit analysis. These findings strengthen conviction that moderator effects do indeed obtain in both samples and cannot be considered spurious.

Note should be taken of the differential participation rates of the two samples: 98 % for the Chinese sample and 74 % for the U.S. sample. Although this difference could suggest a possible source of differential bias, the rate for the Chinese sample is what is extraordinary, and the U.S. sample's participation rate is generally accepted as satisfactory for urban, school-based samples requiring signed parental permission. Finally, of course, this is a report of a cross-sectional study; a longitudinal design will be required for more compelling inference about the influence of protection and risk on adolescent involvement in problem behavior.

Each of these limitations is important to acknowledge as a possible constraint on the inferences that can be drawn from the findings reported. Nevertheless, the study—an exemplification of theory-based cross-national research—has yielded compelling support for the cross-national generality of the protection-risk explanatory model in accounting for adolescent problem behavior. It has also drawn attention to the important role of protective factors as both direct and indirect regulators of problem behavior involvement. A greater focus on the delineation and assessment of protection in future research in this field would be a salutary outcome of the present effort and a significant contribution to the design of more effective intervention initiatives.

Acknowledgments This study was supported by Grant 99202099 from the William T. Grant Foundation. We are grateful to the officials of the school districts involved for their support and cooperation, and especially to Gene Jacquez for his extensive contributions. We are also indebted to Guang Guo for reviewing the questionnaire translation; to Charles M. Judd, Gary H. McClelland, and Jani Little for consultation on data analysis; and to Carissa Low for exceptionally competent assistance in many aspects of the research.

References

Aiken, L. S., & West, S. G. (1991). *Multiple regression: Testing and interpreting interactions.* Newbury Park, CA: Sage.

Alsaker, F. D., & Flammer, A. (1999). *The adolescent experience: European and American adolescents in the 1990s.* Mahwah, NJ: Erlbaum.

Barber, B. K. (1997). Introduction: Adolescent socialization in context—The role of connection, regulation, and autonomy in the family. *Journal of Adolescent Research, 12*, 5–11.

Barber, B. K., & Olsen, J. A. (1997). Socialization in context: Connection, regulation, and autonomy in the family, school, and neighborhood, and with peers. *Journal of Adolescent Research, 12*, 287–315.

Chen, C., Greenberger, E., Farruggia, S., Bush, K., & Dong, Q. (2003). Beyond parents and peers: The role of important non-parental adults (VIPs) in adolescent development in China and the United States. *Psychology in the Schools, 40*, 35–50.

Chen, C., Greenberger, E., Lester, J., Dong, Q., & Guo, M. (1998). A cross-cultural study of family and peer correlates of adolescent misconduct. *Developmental Psychology, 34*, 770–781.

Chen, Y., Dong, Q., & Zhou, H. (1997). Authoritative and authoritarian parenting practices and social and school performance in Chinese children. *International Journal of Behavioral Development, 21*, 855–873.

Cohen, J., & Cohen, P. (1983). *Applied multiple regression/correlation analysis for the behavioral sciences* (2nd ed.). Hillsdale, NJ: Erlbaum.

Costa, F. M., Jessor, R., & Turbin, M. S. (1999). Transition into adolescent problem drinking: The role of psychosocial risk and protective factors. *Journal of Studies on Alcohol, 60*(4), 480–490.

Darling, N., & Steinberg, L. (1993). Parenting style as context: An integrative model. *Psychological Bulletin, 113*, 487–496.

Dong, Q., & Chen, C. (2001). The role of relationships with teachers in adolescent development among a national sample of Chinese urban adolescents. *Chinese Journal of Applied Psychology, 7*(2), 3–10.

Donovan, J. E., & Jessor, R. (1985). Structure of problem behavior in adolescence and young adulthood. *Journal of Consulting and Clinical Psychology, 53*(6), 890–904.

Dornbusch, S., Ritter, P., Leiderman, R., Roberts, D., & Fraleigh, M. (1987). The relation of parenting style to adolescent school performance. *Child Development, 58*, 1244–1257.

Ekblad, S. (1986). Relationships between child-rearing practice and primary school children's functional adjustment in the People's Republic of China. *Scandinavian Journal of Psychology, 27*, 220–230.

Elliott, D. S. (1993). Health-enhancing and health-compromising lifestyles. In S. G. Millstein, A. C. Petersen, & E. O. Nightingale (Eds.), *Promoting the health of adolescents: New directions for the twenty-first century* (pp. 119–145). New York: Oxford University Press.

Felix-Ortiz, M., & Newcomb, M. D. (1992). Risk and protective factors for drug use among Latino and White adolescents. *Hispanic Journal of Behavioral Sciences, 14*, 291–309.

Greenberger, E., Chen, C., Beam, M., Whang, S., & Dong, Q. (2000). The perceived social contexts of adolescents' misconduct: A comparative study of youths in three cultures. *Journal of Research on Adolescence, 10*, 365–388.

Guang-Ren, L. (1997). An investigation of adolescent health from China. *Journal of Adolescent Health, 20*, 306–308.

Hawkins, J. D., Catalano, R. F., & Miller, J. Y. (1992). Risk and protective factors for alcohol and other drug problems in adolescence and early adulthood: Implications for substance abuse prevention. *Psychological Bulletin, 112*, 64–105.

Hesketh, T., Ding, Q. J., & Tomkins, A. (2001). Smoking among youths in China. *American Journal of Public Health, 91*, 1653–1655.

Ho, D. Y. F. (1986). Chinese patterns of socialization: A critical review. In M. H. Bond (Ed.), *The psychology of the Chinese people* (pp. 1–37). New York: Oxford University Press.

Jessor, R. (1998). New perspectives on adolescent risk behavior. In R. Jessor (Ed.), *New perspectives on adolescent risk behavior* (pp. 1–10). New York: Cambridge University Press.
Jessor, R., Donovan, J. E., & Costa, F. M. (1991). *Beyond adolescence: Problem behavior and young adult development*. New York: Cambridge University Press.
Jessor, R., Graves, T. D., Hanson, R. C., & Jessor, S. L. (1968). *Society, personality, and deviant behavior: A study of a tri-ethnic community*. New York: Holt, Rinehart & Winston.
Jessor, R., & Jessor, S. L. (1977). *Problem behavior and psychosocial development: A longitudinal study of youth*. New York: Academic Press.
Jessor, R., Turbin, M. S., & Costa, F. M. (1998a). Protective factors in adolescent health behavior. *Journal of Personality and Social Psychology, 75*(3), 788–800.
Jessor, R., Turbin, M. S., & Costa, F. M. (1998b). Risk and protection in successful outcomes among disadvantaged adolescents. *Applied Developmental Science, 2*, 194–208.
Jessor, R., Van Den Bos, J., Vanderryn, J., Costa, F. M., & Turbin, M. S. (1995). Protective factors in adolescent problem behavior: Moderator effects and developmental change. *Developmental Psychology, 31*(6), 923–933.
Johnston, L. D., O'Malley, P. M., & Bachman, J. G. (2001). *Monitoring the future national survey results on drug use, 1975–2000. Vol. 1: Secondary school students* (NIH Publication No. 01-4924). Bethesda, MD: National Institute on Drug Abuse
Kandel, D. B. (1985). On processes of peer influences in adolescent drug use: A developmental perspective. *Advances in Alcohol & Substance Abuse, 4*, 139–163.
Kelley, M. L. (1992). Cultural differences in child rearing: A comparison of immigrant Chinese and Caucasian American mothers. *Journal of Cross-Cultural Psychology, 23*, 444–455.
Knight, G. P., & Hill, N. E. (1998). Measurement equivalence in research involving minority adolescents. In V. C. McLoyd & L. Steinberg (Eds.), *Studying minority adolescents: Conceptual, methodological, and theoretical issues* (pp. 183–210). Mahwah, NJ: Erlbaum.
Lewin, K. (1931). The conflict between Aristotelian and Galileian modes of thought in contemporary psychology. *Journal of General Psychology, 5*, 141–177.
Li, X., Fang, X., & Stanton, B. (1996). Cigarette smoking among Chinese adolescents and its association with demographic characteristics, social activities, and problem behaviors. *Substance Use & Misuse, 31*, 545–563.
Li, X., Fang, X., Stanton, B., Feigelman, S., & Dong, Q. (1996). The rate and pattern of alcohol consumption among Chinese adolescents. *Journal of Adolescent Health, 19*, 353–361.
Lin, C. C., & Fu, V. R. (1990). A comparison of child-rearing practices among Chinese, immigrant Chinese, and Caucasian-American parents. *Child Development, 61*, 429–433.
McClelland, G. H., & Judd, C. M. (1993). Statistical difficulties of detecting interactions and moderator effects. *Psychological Bulletin, 114*, 376–390.
Oetting, E. R., & Beauvais, F. (1987). Common elements in youth drug abuse: Peer clusters and other psychosocial factors. *Journal of Drug Issues, 17*, 133–151.
Resnick, M. D., Bearman, P. S., Blum, R. W., Bauman, K. E., Harris, K. M., Jones, J., et al. (1997). Protecting adolescents from harm: Findings from the National Longitudinal Study on Adolescent Health. *Journal of the American Medical Association, 278*, 823–832.
Rojek, D. G. (2001). Chinese social control: From shaming to reintegration to "getting rich is glorious". In J. Liu, L. Zhang, & S. E. Messner (Eds.), *Crime and social control in a changing China* (pp. 89–103). Westport, CT: Greenwood Press.
Stacy, A. W., Newcomb, M. D., & Bentler, P. M. (1992). Interactive and higher-order effects of social influences on drug use. *Journal of Health and Social Behavior, 33*, 226–241.
Unger, J. B., Yan, L., Chen, X., Jiang, X., Azen, S., Qian, G., et al. (2001). Adolescent smoking in Wuhan, China: Baseline data from the Wuhan Smoking Prevention Trial. *American Journal of Preventive Medicine, 21*, 162–169.
Unger, J. B., Yan, L., Shakib, S., Rohrbach, L. A., Chen, X., Qian, G., et al. (2002). Peer influences and access to cigarettes as correlates of adolescent smoking: A cross-cultural comparison of Wuhan, China, and California. *Preventive Medicine, 34*, 476–484.
Wills, T. A., Vaccaro, D., & McNamara, G. (1992). The role of life events, family support, and competence in adolescent substance use: A test of vulnerability and protective factors. *American Journal of Community Psychology, 20*, 349–374.

Wong, L. (1995). Reforming welfare and relief–socializing the state's burden. In L.Wong, & S. MacPherson (Eds.), *Social change and social policy in contemporary China* (pp. 50–69).
Wong, L., & Mok, K. (1995). The reform and the changing social context. In L. Wong & S. MacPherson (Eds.), *Social change and social policy in contemporary China* (pp. 1–26). Aldershot, England: Avebury.
Wu, D. H. (1981). Child abuse in Taiwan. In J. E. Korbin (Ed.), *Child abuse and neglect: Cross-cultural perspectives* (pp. 139–165). Los Angeles: University of California Press.
Ye, G. (1997). Health promotion of adolescents. *Collegium Antropologicum, 21*, 93–100.
Zhang, L., & Messner, S. F. (1996). School attachment and official delinquency status in the People's Republic of China. *Sociological Forum, 11*, 285–303.
Zhang, L., Wang, W., Zhao, Q., & Vartainen, E. (2000). Psychosocial predictors of smoking among secondary school students in Henan, China. *Health Education Research, 15*, 415–422.
Zhimin, L., Weihua, Z., Zhi, L., Yue, M., Zhiji, C., & Jiaqi, C. (2001). The use of psychoactive substances among adolescent students in an area in the south-west of China. *Addiction, 96*, 247–250.

Chapter 11
Problem Behavior Theory and Adolescent Pro-Social Behavior

Richard Jessor and Mark S. Turbin

Introduction

In this study, we investigate the different roles played by protective factors and risk factors—and by particular protective and risk factors—when the concern is with accounting for adolescent problem behavior versus when the concern is with accounting for adolescent pro-social behavior. Recent decades have seen a burgeoning of interest in the role of protective and risk factors in accounting for variation in adolescent problem behavior (e.g., Jessor, 1991; Hawkins, Catalano, & Miller, 1992; Luthar & Cicchetti, 2000; Jessor et al., 1995; Jessor, Turbin, & Costa, 1998a & b; Jessor et al., 2003; Jessor, 2014; Bernat, Oakes, Pettingell, & Resnick, 2012). Despite substantial support for their explanatory usefulness, there has been considerable ambiguity in how their meaning has been conceptualized and their measurement operationalized by different investigators. The application in the present study of the protective and risk factor constructs of Problem Behavior Theory (Jessor, 1991, 2014; Jessor et al., 1995) is an effort to advance analytic understanding in this domain of inquiry. The very same protection and risk model is used, in this article, to account for variation in *both* problem behavior and pro-social behavior. This approach, contrasting an analysis of a problem behavior criterion with an analysis of a pro-social behavior criterion, should yield results that illuminate the different

---

Reprinted with permission from:
Jessor, R., & Turbin, M. S. (2014). Parsing protection and risk for problem behavior versus pro-social behavior among US and Chinese adolescents. *Journal of Youth and Adolescence, 43*(7), 1037–1051.

R. Jessor (✉)
Institute of Behavioral Science, University of Colorado at Boulder, Boulder, CO, USA
e-mail: jessor@Colorado.edu

M.S. Turbin
Kalispell, MT, USA

R. Jessor, *The Origins and Development of Problem Behavior Theory*,
Advancing Responsible Adolescent Development,
DOI 10.1007/978-3-319-40886-6_11

roles played by particular protective and risk factors in the two analyses and also document the *promotive* function of protection.

The risk factor construct, borrowed from epidemiology, implies a greater likelihood of occurrence of problem behavior, while the protective factor construct is invoked to account for a diminished likelihood of occurrence of problem behavior, either as a direct effect or by buffering the impact of exposure to risk. In most of the problem behavior literature, however, when both constructs are brought to bear, it is usually to account for variation in problem behavior alone, and to use that account to suggest approaches for preventing or decreasing problem behavior involvement. What has been omitted in much of the problem behavior research has been a recognition that protective factors do not simply protect against risk and, therefore, against involvement in problem behavior, but that they also have promotive properties and can increase involvement in pro-social behavior. One of the aims of the present study is to demonstrate the positive relationship of protective factors to pro-social behavior involvement.

Also contributing to conceptual ambiguity has been the connotative meaning of the term "protective," an adjective that implies protecting against something, here against risk. Even when the effect of protective factors as moderators or buffers is acknowledged, the emphasis is generally on their reducing the impact of risk, e.g., "Protective factors are those that modify the effects of risk in a positive direction." (Luthar & Cicchetti, 2000, p. 858). But that is a limitation that leaves open the question of what function protective factors might have *independent of the presence of risk.* Conceptualizing protective factors as *promotive* of pro-social behavior, as well as preventive of problem behavior, provides them with a function that expands their explanatory contribution to variation in adolescent behavior, both problem and pro-social. And involvement in pro-social behavior itself can, theoretically, serve as a protective factor against engaging in problem behavior. It is this latter conceptualization of protection, as both preventive and promotive, that has been relied upon in this research.

The promotive function of protective factors has, of course, been the main emphasis of the positive youth development approach to adolescence with its focus on developmental assets and competencies of young people (e.g., Benson, 1997; Lerner & Benson, 2003). In seeking to counter the emphasis on youth as "problems," however, research on positive youth development has at times ignored problem behavior or just assumed that problem behaviors would diminish as protective factors are brought to bear, even without specific attention to risk reduction. Important efforts have been made to bridge this divide between research on problem behaviors and research on positive development (e.g., Guerra & Bradshaw, 2008; Hilliard et al., 2014; Phelps et al., 2007), but the promotive function of protective factors has not yet been fully assimilated in most problem behavior research. The present study, in engaging *both* problem behavior and pro-social behavior, aims to illuminate the promotive role of protective factors on positive behavior as well as their preventive role on problem behavior.

Further conceptual ambiguity derives from the practice of some investigators to specify protective and risk factors at the descriptive-level, the level that Lewin (1935), borrowing concepts from genetics, termed the phenotypic level, whereas others do so at the explanatory or genotypic level. For example, to consider a "mentor" for an at-risk adolescent as a protective factor would be an example of a descriptive-level or phenotypic designation; at the explanatory or genotypic level, what is actually protective are those behavioral processes that underlie what mentoring usually entails, namely, the modeling of pro-social behavior, the provision of social support, and the exercise of informal social controls. As another example, the descriptive-level risk factor, "neighborhood disorganization," entails at the genotypic level such risk factors as pervasive models for problem behavior, ready opportunity for engaging in problem behavior (via the presence of gangs), and personal vulnerability to risk exposure. In the present study, risk and protective factors are specified at the explanatory or genotypic level rather than at the descriptive or phenotypic level.

Finally, various investigators have determined which variables constitute protective factors and which constitute risk factors largely post hoc, that is, depending on the outcome of research: if a predictor variable relates in a positive direction to problem behavior in the empirical findings it is specified as a risk factor, and if it relates in a negative direction it is specified as a protective factor (e.g., Bernat et al., 2012; Blum et al., 2003; Pardini, Loeber, Farrington, & Stouthamer-Loeber, 2012; Simantov, Schoen, & Klein, 2000). Without some a priori basis—theoretical or even common sense—such an entirely empirical and post hoc approach is unlikely to advance understanding. Nor is the often-related approach of specifying protection and risk as simply the opposite ends of a given dimension; for example, if high religiosity is identified as a protective factor then low religiosity is, therefore, deemed a risk factor (e.g., Herrenkohl, Lee, & Hawkins, 2012; Lösel & Farrington, 2012). Lost in this latter approach, of course, are the unique conceptual properties that protection and risk have and the explanatory value of retaining their conceptual independence which permits exploring their interaction or moderator effects. In the present study, protective and risk factors are specified theoretically rather than empirically, and their relationship is posited, theoretically, as orthogonal.

Problem Behavior Theory

The bulk of problem behavior research engaging protective and risk factor constructs has focused on the various manifestations of adolescent problem or risk behaviors, ranging across delinquency, marijuana and other illicit drug use, early and unprotected sex, tobacco and alcohol involvement, violence, school dropout, risky driving, and more recently such practices as gambling and cyber bullying. Clearly a very diverse array phenotypically, but all related because of the transgression of social or legal norms that is involved or the failure to fulfill normal social role expectations, e.g., at school or at work. Since its inception a half century ago (Jessor, Graves, Hanson, & Jessor, 1968; Jessor, 2014), Problem Behavior Theory has been applied to most of these problem behavior domains, not only by our Colorado group but by other investigators in the US and across the globe (e.g.,

Costa et al., 2005; Jessor, 2014; Madkour, Farhat, Halpern, Godeau, & Gabhainn, 2010; Ndugwa et al., 2010; Vazsonyi et al., 2008, 2010). Revised and elaborated over the years since 1968, Problem Behavior Theory is now constituted of sets of theoretically specified protective factors and risk factors, in both the individual adolescent and the social context, organized to account for variation in both problem behavior and pro-social behavior in adolescence.

Four protective factors that theoretically have a direct influence on the likelihood of occurrence of behavior have been articulated: models for pro-social behavior (Models Protection); informal social and personal controls against problem behavior (Controls Protection); social support for pro-social behavior (Support Protection); and actual engagement in pro-social behavior (Behavior Protection). Each protective factor captures an underlying process, e.g., social modeling, that, theoretically, can regulate or constrain problem behavior or promote the occurrence of pro-social behavior. Four risk factors that theoretically have a direct influence on the likelihood of occurrence of behavior have also been specified: models for problem behavior (Models Risk); opportunity to engage in problem behavior (Opportunity Risk); vulnerability for engaging in problem behavior (Vulnerability Risk); and actual engagement in problem behavior (Behavior Risk). The theoretical rationale for each of these constructs as protective factors or as risk factors was described by Jessor (1991) and Jessor et al., (2003) and, most recently, was elaborated in Jessor (2014). In short, each represents an influence on or determinant of behavior, both problem and pro-social. Their operational definitions in the current study are described in the "Methods" section below. In Problem Behavior Theory, beyond their having direct effects on preventing or reducing problem behavior involvement, protective factors are also theoretically specified as having effects as moderators or buffers of the impact of exposure to risk, operationalized as significant interactions of the protective factors with the risk factors in regression analyses. Figure 11.1 illustrates the theoretical framework of protection and risk, and of their interaction, as implemented and tested in the present study.

The relative explanatory importance of the different protective and risk factors has been a topic of interest in a variety of studies. The protective factor of "support," or the related notion of "connectedness" in the literature, has often been given a salient role as a protective factor against problem behavior (Barber, 1997; Barber & Olsen, 1997); there has also been an emphasis in the literature on "controls"—rules, regulations, sanctions-as a protective factor against problem behavior, sometimes defined as parental rules and sanctions, sometimes as parental monitoring and knowledge (Kerr & Stattin, 2000; Piko & Kovacs, 2010) and Barber and Xia (2013) has further differentiated parental control into behavioral control and psychological control. In our own prior research, Costa et al., (2005) found that Controls Protection was a pre-eminent protective factor in both direct and moderator effects on adolescent problem behavior, whereas Support Protection played a much more limited role. It was speculated then that: "Support Protection could well play a larger role when the criterion is positive, pro-social behavior, and that possibility remains a matter for further inquiry" (p. 81).That further inquiry is a key aspect of the present research.

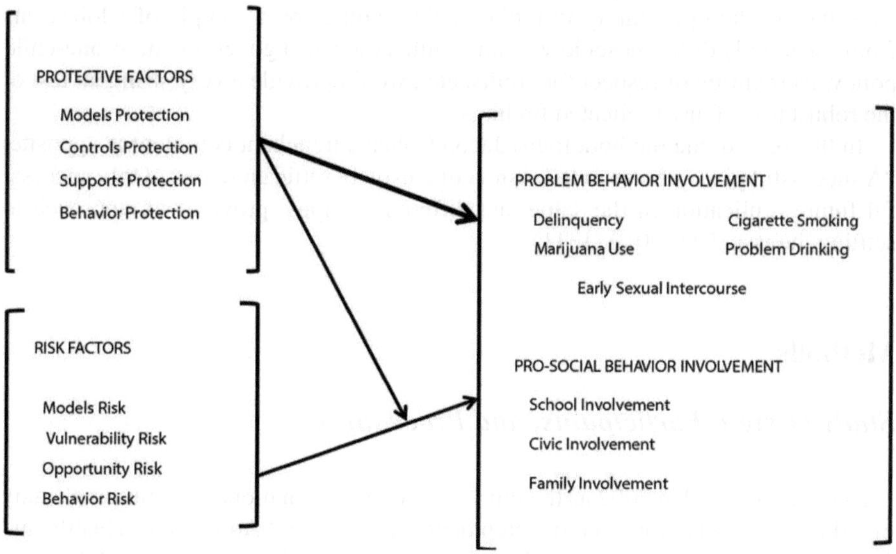

Fig. 11.1 Problem Behavior Theory explanatory framework

The Current Study

The main aim of this study is to examine the applicability of the Problem Behavior Theory framework of protection and risk to *both* problem and pro-social behavior and, in so doing, to illuminate the different roles played by protection and risk, and by the various protective and risk factors, when applied to the two different, even opposing, behavioral outcome criteria. It was expected, for example, that Controls Protection, while an important protective factor against problem behavior, might play a less significant role in accounting for variation in pro-social behavior since its function is largely regulatory rather than promotive; further, it was expected that Models Risk, a major risk factor for problem behavior, might be less important in relationship to pro-social behavior since it represents models for problem behavior, not for positive behavior. As noted above, it was also expected that Support Protection should be more influential for pro-social behavior variation than for problem behavior variation because it represents support for positive behavior. Establishing such differential roles for particular protective and risk factors could have important implications for those interventions seeking to reduce problem behavior versus those seeking to promote or enhance pro-social behavior. This was the secondary aim that animated this study.

Data from a large cross-national, comparative study of adolescents in China and the US (Jessor et al., 2003, 2010; Jessor, Turbin, & Costa, 2010; Costa et al., 2005; Turbin et al., 2006) provided the opportunity to pursue these aims. Having data from two different samples of adolescents permits an immediate replication that can strengthen whatever inferences are drawn from the findings. And, in the present case, having the opportunity to replicate the findings on a sample of adolescents from a markedly different society, China, with its socialist government, its one-child policy, its tradition of respect for adults, etc., would provide a very stringent test of the robustness of any replicated findings.

In this regard, the methodologist Jacob Cohen's trenchant comment is apposite: "A successful piece of research doesn't conclusively settle an issue.... Only successful future replication in the same and different settings. provides an approach to settling the issue" (1990, p. 1311).

Methods

Study Design, Participants, and Procedures

Data were collected in 2002 as the third wave of a cross-national, longitudinal study of adolescent behavior and development. A 32-page "Adolescent Health and Development Questionnaire" (AHDQ) was administered to samples of adolescents in schools in Beijing, China and in a large urban area in the Rocky Mountain region of the US. The AHDQ is the most recent version of a theory-derived questionnaire developed over the past several decades for use in both local and national sample studies (e.g., Jessor et al., 1995). Content of the AHDQ is logically derived from the constructs in Problem Behavior Theory. The questionnaire assesses a broad range of pro-social and problem behaviors, as well as psychosocial and behavioral protective factors and risk factors in the individual adolescent (values, beliefs, attitudes, expectations, and behaviors) and in the four social contexts of daily adolescent life: family, peers, school, and neighborhood. The full AHDQ with exact wording of items and response categories can be found at: http://www.colorado.edu/ibs/jessor/questionnaires/questionnaire_ahdq3.pdf.

Before the study began, the AHDQ was translated into Chinese and then back-translated into English by members of the Chinese research team. The translation and the back-translation were then reviewed in detail by a Chinese social scientist at the University of North Carolina. In addition, the Chinese language version of the AHDQ was reviewed by a native Chinese student at the University of Colorado, Boulder, and the back-translation was reviewed by members of the US research team. On the basis of these multiple reviews, a few instances where the meaning may have been compromised in translation were communicated to the Chinese team, and the Chinese version of the AHDQ was revised accordingly. Both of the Chinese-speaking reviewers in the US found the Chinese translation of the AHDQ to be very well done, and the agreed-upon equivalence of the two versions undergirds the appropriateness of comparisons between the Chinese and US samples. Similarity across the US and Chinese samples of alpha reliability coefficients and of bivariate validity coefficients for a large number of measures in the AHDQ has been shown in an earlier study of the Wave-1 data (Jessor et al., 2003); such similarity provides further support for the inference of "meaning equivalence" of the two versions (see Knight & Hill, 1998).

In Wave-3 of the study, 2533 students now in grades 9, 10, and 11 (76 % of the Wave-1 participants) took part— 1392 in the Chinese sample (87 % of the Chinese Wave-1 sample) and 1141 in the US sample (71 % of the US Wave-1 sample). (For details about selection of schools and of classes within schools, see Jessor et al., 2003) Active parental consent and personal consent were required. Letters describing the study to the parents and adolescents were distributed to the sampled students, and signed consent forms were returned to teachers. Study participants filled out the questionnaire at school in large-group administration sessions proctored by research staff. Each participant received a token payment—$10 in the US; $2, plus a gift to each school, in Beijing. In both countries, about half the Wave-3 participants are female (50 % in China; 56 % in the US), and about a third were in grades 9 (32 and 31 %, respectively), 10 (35 %), and 11 (33 and 34 %, respectively). In the US, 43 % of the sample self-described as Hispanic, 30 % as African American, 22 % as White, 4 % as Asian American, and 1 % as American Indian. Nearly all (96 %) of the Chinese participants are of Han descent.

Adolescent Problem Behavior Involvement

The Multiple Problem Behavior Index (MPBI) assesses overall level of involvement in five different types of adolescent-reported problem behavior: (1) delinquent behavior, ten items including theft, vandalism, and physical aggression (α=.84, US; .82, China); (2) cigarette smoking, based on self-reports of frequency and amount of smoking in the past month and in the past year (α=.79, US; .84, China); (3) problem drinking, based on respondents' reports of frequency of drunkenness and frequency of high-volume drinking (4 or more drinks per occasion) α=.69, US; .64, China); (4) marijuana use (one item, frequency of use in the past 6 months); and (5) sexual experience (a single item reporting any sexual intercourse history). Reported prevalence of marijuana use in the China sample was so low (6 participants, or 0.5 % of Wave-3 responses) that the MPBI (and also the related measures of protective and risk factors described below) was computed for the China sample excluding items about marijuana. Measures of the five components of the index (four components in the China sample) were transformed into *T*-scores (mean of 50 and standard deviation of 10) within each sample and averaged. In both countries, as would be expected, mean scores on this MPBI measure are significantly higher for older participants than for younger ones and, in China only, males have significantly higher MPBI scores than do females.

Adolescent Pro-social Behavior Involvement

The Multiple Pro-social Behavior Index (MPSBI) assesses involvement in three different types of adolescent-reported pro-social behavior: (1) activities with family, five items assessing the frequency in the past 6 months of activities with parents, such as going out to a movie, working together on a hobby or project, or going on a family hike ($\alpha = .81$ both samples); (2) involvement in school and community activities, six items assessing participation and time spent in school clubs (except sports), community or church groups, and volunteer work ($\alpha = .75$ both samples); and (3) a single item assessing hours per week spent doing homework. The MPSBI is the sum of z-scores of those three pro-social behavior measures.

Protection and Risk

A description of each Wave-3 measure is presented in Table 11.1. Protective factors and risk factors were assessed by multiple items for the most part, and scores for each measure were computed as averages of equally weighted z-scored items. For the social-contextual measures, the adolescent respondent characterized protection and risk as perceived in the social settings navigated in his/her everyday life—family, peers, school, and neighborhood; thus, all of the social context measures in the AHDQ are perceived context measures.

The protective and risk factor measures assessed the four kinds of protective factors (Models Protection, Controls Protection, Support Protection, and Behavior Protection) and the four kinds of risk factors (Models Risk, Opportunity Risk, Vulnerability Risk, and Behavior Risk) specified in Problem Behavior Theory. Although an effort was made to measure every construct in every context, limitations on the length of the questionnaire made it necessary to omit measures of some of the contexts.

Measures of Protection

Models Protection. Models Protection was assessed in two contexts, family and peers. A 20-item scale of Models Protection ($\alpha = .83$ and .84 for the US and China samples, respectively) asks about parent and peer involvement in various conventional organizations and pro-social pastimes [e.g., "Does either of your parents take part" in community groups (specified to encompass organizations relevant to each country, like the Parent-Teacher Organization in the US, or the equivalent organization in China), or volunteer work (like at a hospital in the US, or in a "welfare service" in China)], and in health-enhancing behaviors (e.g., "How many of your friends pay attention to eating a healthy diet?").

Controls Protection. Controls Protection was measured in each of the four social contexts and also at the individual-level. Controls Protection is a 43-item scale (40 items in China; $\alpha = .92$ and .91 for the US and China samples, respectively) that assesses strictness of parental rules (e.g., about being home by a certain time at night), parental monitoring of the adolescent (e.g., "Do your parents make sure they know who you're spending your time with?"); parental sanctions (e.g., "If your parents knew that you had shoplifted something from a store, would you get in trouble for it?"); perceived friends' controls against social transgressions

Table 11.1 Protective and risk factor composite measures, component subscales, and Wave-3 alpha reliabilities

Measure [no. of items, (US, China if different)]	Cronbach's alpha	
	US sample	China sample
Protective Factors		
Models Protection (20)	.83	.84
Parent Models for Conventional Behavior (3)		
Parent Models for Health Behavior (8)		
Friends Models for Conventional Behavior (5)		
Friends Models for Health Behavior (4)		
Controls Protection (43, 40)	.92	.91
Attitudinal Intolerance of Deviance (10)[a]		
Parent Sanctions (5, 4)		
Family Controls (8)		
Peer Controls (4)		
Friends Disapproval (3, 2)		
School Controls (3)		
Student Disapproval (4)		
Neighborhood Controls (3)		
Neighborhood Disapproval (3, 2)		
Support Protection (16)	.85	.86
Family Support (7)		
Friends Support (2)		
Teacher Support (4)		
Neighborhood Support (3)		
Behavior Protection Index—MPSBI (3)[a]	–	–
Family Activities (5)		
School and Community Activities (6)		
Hours/Week Doing Homework (1)		
Risk Factors		
Models Risk (18, 15)	.83	.78
Family Models for Risk Behavior (1)		
Peer Models for Risk Behavior (8, 7)		
School Models for Risk Behavior (6, 5)		
Neighborhood Models for Substance Use (3, 2)		
Opportunity Risk (4, 3)	.58	.71
Availability of Cigarettes at Home (1)		
Availability of Alcohol at Home (1)		
Availability of Alcohol in the Neighborhood (1)		
Availability of Marijuana in the Neighborhood (1, US Only)		
Vulnerability Risk (19)[a]	.88	.84
Depression (3)		
Low Expectations for Academic Achievement (4)		
Low Perceived Life Chances (5)		
Low Self-Esteem (7)		
Behavior Risk Index—MPBI (5, 4)[a]	–	–
Delinquent Behavior (10)		
Cigarette Smoking (2)		
High-Volume Drinking (2)		
Sexual Intercourse (1)		
Marijuana Use (1, US Only)		

Alpha reliability is not meaningful for the behavior indexes

[a]Individual-level measures

(e.g., "If you were going to do something that most people think is wrong, would your friends try to stop you?"); perceived friends' disapproval of risk behaviors (e.g., "How do most of your friends feel about someone your age drinking alcohol?"); perceived institutional controls against student misbehavior (e.g., "In your school, how strict are the rules about student behavior in class, in the halls, and on the school grounds?"); perceived student disapproval of student misbehavior such as cheating and vandalism (e.g., "What do most of the students at your school think about kids who damage school property?"); perceived neighborhood disapproval of teenage transgression e.g., smoking, drinking, and vandalism (e.g., "How do you think most of the adults in your neighborhood feel about someone your age smoking cigarettes or drinking alcohol?"); and perceived neighborhood controls against adolescent misbehavior (e.g., "If adults in your neighborhood saw kids doing something wrong or getting in trouble, would they tell the parents about it?"). And at the individual-level, Controls Protection was measured by 10 items that assess attitudinal intolerance of normative transgression (e.g., "How wrong do you think it is to cheat on tests or homework?").

Support Protection. Support Protection was measured in all four contexts by 16 items assessing perceived social support (α=.85, US; .86, China). Support Protection includes seven items in the family context (e.g., "Are your parents interested in what you think and how you feel?"); two items in the peer context (e.g., "When you have personal problems, do your friends try to understand and let you know they care?"); four items in the school context (e.g., "Do teachers at your school try to help students when they are having problems?"); and three items in the neighborhood context (e.g., "In your neighborhood, do people help each other out and look after each other?").

Behavior Protection. Behavior Protection was measured by the Multiple Pro-social Behavior Index, described above, in the analyses of problem behavior variation. Since it is an index rather than a scale, an alpha is not calculated.

Measures of Risk

Models Risk. Models Risk was measured in all four contexts. Models Risk (α=.83, US; .78, China) comprises one family context item ("Does anyone in your close family smoke cigarettes?"); and 17 items (14 items in the China sample) across the other three social contexts, assessing social models for a variety of risk behaviors (e.g., school dropout, delinquent behavior, unhealthy diet, cigarette smoking, alcohol use). Example items are: "How many of your friends have dropped out of school or are thinking about it?"; "How many of the students at your school get into fights?"; and "How much drinking is there among adults in your neighborhood, as far as you know?"

Opportunity Risk. Opportunity Risk was measured in two contexts. Opportunity Risk (α=.58, US; .71, China) comprises four items (three items in the China sample) that assess perceived availability of cigarettes and alcohol in the home, and perceived availability of alcohol and marijuana in the neighborhood.

Vulnerability Risk. Vulnerability Risk was assessed by a multiple-item measure of personal vulnerability. The 19 items in this scale ($\alpha=.88$, US; .84, China) all measure personal vulnerability risk, including depression (three items, e.g., "In the past 6 months, have you just felt really down about things?"); limited perceived chances for success in life (five items, e.g., "What are the chances that you will have a job that pays well?"); low expectations for school achievement (four items, e.g., "How sure are you that you will get at least a B average this year?"); and low self-esteem (seven items, e.g., "On the whole, how satisfied are you with yourself?").

Behavior Risk. Behavior Risk was measured by the Multiple Problem Behavior Index (MPBI), described above, in analyses of pro-social behavior variation.

In general, the multiple-item scales used to assess protection and risk in the four social contexts and at the individual-level have good scale properties (Table 11.1), although the alphas for Opportunity Risk were lower (.58, US; .71, China). Overall, then, the complete set of measures provides, with acceptable reliability and with well-established construct validity from earlier studies, a theoretically comprehensive assessment of protection and risk at the individual-level and across the four social contexts.

Correlations among the psychosocial protective and risk factors are shown in Table 11.2, separately for each gender within each country sample. As expected, in each subgroup, the protective factors are positively related among themselves, as are the risk factors, and each protective factor is negatively related to each risk factor. The strongest correlations are among the protective factors. In particular, Controls Protection and Support Protection are correlated around .60 for each subgroup.

Table 11.2 Bivariate correlations among and between protective and risk factor measures

Measure	Models Protection	Controls Protection	Support Protection	Models Risk	Vulnerability Risk	Opportunity Risk
US sample						
Models Protection	–	.46	.42	−.22	−.38	−.20
Controls Protection	.50	–	.62	−.47	−.42	−.42
Support Protection	.57	.63	–	−.29	−.52	−.27
Models Risk	−.39	−.55	−.47	–	.22	.45
Vulnerability Risk	−.36	−.39	−.49	.30	–	.15
Opportunity Risk	−.23	−.45	−.27	.47	.08	–
China sample						
Models Protection	–	.34	.51	−.21	−.33	−.21
Controls Protection	.46	–	.58	−.51	−.33	−.23
Support Protection	.53	.58	–	−.38	−.45	−.17
Models Risk	−.30	−.41	−.35	–	.24	.21
Vulnerability Risk	−.35	−.28	−.43	.23	–	.12
Opportunity Risk	−.28	−.29	−.22	.27	.13	–

Correlations for males are in the upper triangle, for females in the lower triangle
All correlations are significant at $p<.05$

Method of Analysis

The analytic procedure used in the research is hierarchical multiple regression testing protection and risk main effects and their interactions. All analyses were run separately for the China sample and the US sample. Since standardized regression coefficients are inappropriate with interaction terms (Aiken & West, 1991, pp. 40-47), all predictor measures were standardized to make the unstandardized regression coefficients comparable to one another. Because intra-class correlations were negligible, ranging from .02 China to .03 US, indicating that students' responses on the criterion measures can be treated as independent observations, multilevel modeling was not used.

Measures of socio-demographic characteristics were entered at Step 1 of each hierarchical regression analysis to control for the effects of gender, grade in school, intact family (i.e., families that include both biological parents versus families missing at least one biological parent), and socioeconomic status [average of father's job level (a Hollingshead-type rating) and father's and mother's educational attainment; for homes with no father, average of mother's job level and educational level].

Results

Results are presented in the following order. First, we examine the protective and risk factor explanatory account of variation in problem behavior (the MPBI criterion measure) in Wave-3 of the study. The participants are now in mid-adolescence (age 15–17), and the current findings predicting problem behavior can be compared with those previously reported from the Wave-1 analyses (Jessor et al., 2003) when the participants were in early adolescence (age 13–15). Next, we examine whether the same model, applied first to account for variation in problem behavior, is also useful in explaining variation in prosocial behavior (the MPSBI criterion measure). The contrasting analyses can reveal whether the roles played by protection and risk, and by particular protective and risk factors, differ when accounting for problem behavior versus pro-social behavior—the key concerns of the present study.

Applying Problem Behavior Theory to Account for Adolescent Problem Behavior (MPBI)

The complement of protective factors used in the present analysis was enlarged over that used in the Wave-1 analyses by the inclusion of the measure of Behavior Protection (MPSBI), now part of the expanded theoretical model (Jessor, 2014). Regression results are shown in Table 11.3. Also shown in the first column for each sample in Table 11.3, are the bivariate correlations of the four protective factors

Table 11.3 Hierarchical regression of the Multiple Problem Behavior Index (MPBI) on protective factors and risk factors in the US and China: Wave-3

Step		US			China		
		r	b^a, final step	ΔR^2	r	b^a, final step	ΔR^2
1	Socio-demographic Background			.03			.08
	Gender (f = 1, m = −1)	.01	.26		−.26***	−.80***	
	Grade in School	.14***	.57**		.09***	.28	
	Intact Family	−.10***	−.50		−.05*	−.15	
	Socioeconomic Status	.01	.27**		−.06*	.24	
2	Protective Factors[b]			.31			.18
	Models Protection	−.28***	.25		−.05*	.92	
	Controls Protection	−.57***	−2.29***		−.48***	−2.04***	
	Support Protection	−.40***	−.02		−.27***	−.06	
	Behavior Protection	−.27***	−.46*		−.08**	.09	
3	Risk Factors			.09			.07
	Models Risk	.55***	2.22***		.45***	1.95***	
	Vulnerability Risk	.30***	.48*		.17***	.47**	
	Opportunity Risk	.37***	.52**		.10***	−.08	
4	Protection-by-Risk Interactions			.05			.06
	Controls Protection × Models Risk		−1.28***			−1.25***	
	Controls Protection × Vulnerability Risk					−.52***	
	Total R^2			.48			.39

N = 1087 (US), 1368 (China). Only significant interactions are included in the final model
*$p \leq .05$; ** $p \leq .01$; *** $p \leq .001$. All ΔR^2 and R^2 values are significant at $p \leq .001$
[a]Unstandardized regression weights of standardized predictor measures; standardized weights are inappropriate with interaction terms (see Aiken & West, 1991, pp. 40–47)
[b]Variance accounted for uniquely by protective factors = .08*** in each sample

with the MPBI criterion; all are significant in the theoretically expected negative direction for both country samples. Of particular interest is the negative correlation of the Behavior Protection measure, the MPSBI, with the problem behavior criterion measure, the MPBI; while significant in both country samples (r = −.27, US; −.08, China), the relationship is small indicating relative independence of the two outcome criteria in the present study. Correlations of the three risk factors with the MPBI outcome criterion are also all significant and in the theoretically expected positive direction for both country samples. These bivariate correlations contribute to the construct validity of the protective and risk factor measures.

At Step 1 of the regressions, the socio-demographic control measures account for a small but significant portion of variance in both country samples. The addition at Step 2 of the protective factors adds a substantial increment to the account, 31 % for the US sample and 18 % for the China sample. Entry of the risk factors at Step 3 adds another significant increment in variance accounted for, 9 % for the US sample and 7 % for the China sample. Finally, at Step 4, there are two significant interactions (of the 12 tested: four protective factors-by-three risk factors) and they add another increment in variance accounted for, 5 % in the US sample and 6 % in the China sample. The total R^2 reaches a substantial 48 % of variance in the US sample and 39 % in the China sample. The applicability of the Problem Behavior Theory framework for explaining involvement in problem behavior, the MPBI, in mid-adolescence is strongly supported in both country samples by these findings.

In light of the study's main objective, it is especially important to take note of the pattern of relative importance among the protective factors and among the risk factors shown by their regression coefficients in Table 11.3. With respect to the protective factors, Controls Protection is the strongest protective factor in both countries and, in China, it is the only protective factor that is significant in the final model. In the US sample, although Behavior Protection is also a significant protective factor, its regression coefficient is only a fifth that of Controls Protection. What is noteworthy in this pattern of regression coefficients is that neither Models Protection nor Support Protection has a significant regression coefficient in the final model in either country sample.

Among the risk factors, the strongest predictor in Table 11.3 is Models Risk. Although the other two risk factors are significant in the US sample and one of them, Vulnerability Risk, is also significant in the China sample, their *b* coefficients are about one-fourth the magnitude of the Models Risk regression coefficient. As shown in Table 11.3, the risk factors entered at Step 3 added 9 and 7 % unique variance. Since the protective factors entered earlier at Step 2 included any variance shared with the risk factors, the order of entry was reversed for the protective and risk factors, in a supplementary regression analysis, to determine the unique variance of the protective factors. In that analysis, the protective factors accounted uniquely for 8 % of variance in each country sample, beyond that accounted for by the socio-demographic and risk measures. Thus, the protective factors and the risk factors accounted uniquely for about equal proportions of the variance in problem behavior involvement, the MPBI, in both country samples.

Further support for the pre-eminent role of Controls Protection in accounting for variation in problem behavior is the fact that it is the only protective factor that significantly moderates risk, Models Risk in the US sample, and both Models Risk and Vulnerability Risk in the China sample, and the magnitude of the interaction effects in both samples is large for field studies (see McClelland & Judd, 1993). The moderator effect of Controls Protection on Models Risk means that the impact of Models Risk on problem behavior is attenuated by higher levels of Controls Protection. Fig. 11.2 illustrates the significant moderator effect of Controls Protection on Models Risk in both country samples; indeed, in the China sample, the line from Low Models Risk to High Models Risk is almost flat under high protection. Since only one of the twelve interactions tested was significant in the US sample and only two in the China sample, concern about Type 1 error could arise. Countering that concern is the evidence that the Controls Protection × Models Risk interaction is significant in both samples, i.e., it is already a replicated finding in this study. In

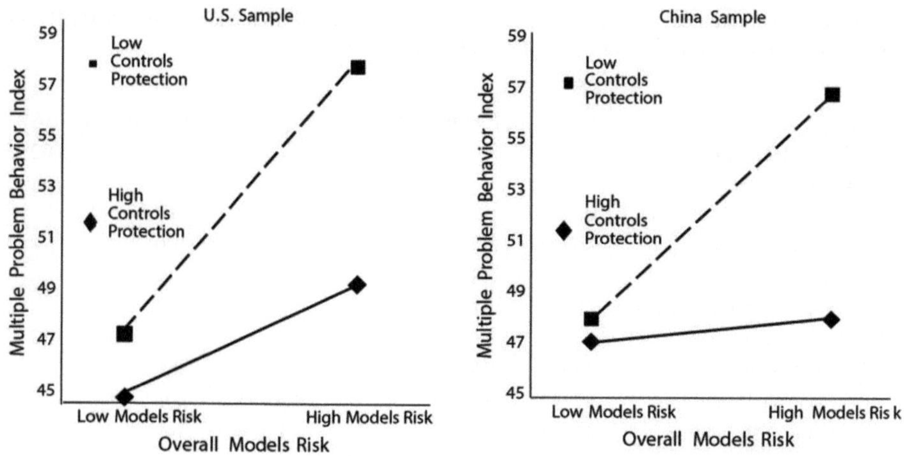

Fig. 11.2 Moderator effect of Controls Protection on Models Risk in US and China samples

addition, it is the same interaction that has emerged in earlier waves of this study, and it is also the same interaction that has emerged in studies by other investigators with other adolescent samples, e.g., adolescents in northern Italy (Ciairano et al., 2009). Finally, the same interaction emerges in the analysis of the pro-social behavior criterion, the MPSBI, for the China sample in the present study.

Applying Problem Behavior Theory to Account for Adolescent Pro-social Behavior (MPSBI)

In this analysis of pro-social behavior involvement, the same protective and risk factor measures were used as were used in the analysis of problem behavior involvement, except that now the MPSBI is the outcome criterion measure to be predicted and the MPBI is now employed as a risk factor, individual-level Behavior Risk. Regression results are shown in Table 11.4.

Again, bivariate correlations of the protective and risk factor measures with the MPSBI in the first column of Table 11.4 show the theoretically expected positive relationships of the protective factors and negative relationships of the risk factors with the MPSBI criterion, contributing to the construct validity of the measures. In general, the correlations of the protective factors are larger than those of the risk factors. The socio-demographic background measures entered at Step 1 of the hierarchical regression account for significant variance, but smaller in the China sample (2 %) than in the US sample (10 %). The entry of the three protective factor measures (models, controls, support) at Step 2 accounted for substantial variance in each sample (22 %, US; 12 %, China). What is especially noteworthy is that both the Models Protection measure and the Support Protection measure, neither of which

Table 11.4 Hierarchical regression of the Multiple Pro-social Behavior Index (MPSBI) on protective factors and risk factors in the US and China: Wave-3

Step		US			China		
		r	*b*[a], final step	ΔR^2	*r*	*b*[a], final step	ΔR^2
1	Socio-demographic Background			.10			.02
	Gender (f=1, m=−1)	.03	.12*		.05*	.11*	
	Grade in School	−.08**	.02		−.06*	−.06	
	Intact Family	.15***	.44***		−.01	−.12	
	Socioeconomic Status	.27***	.21***		.11***	.10*	
2	Protective Factors[b]			.22			.12
	Models Protection	.44***	.43***		.32***	.38***	
	Controls Protection	.37***	.14*		.20***	−.08	
	Support Protection	.45***	.38***		.32***	.34***	
3	Risk Factors			.03			.006
	Models Risk	−.23***	−.02		−.16***	−.06	
	Vulnerability Risk	−.41***	−.32***		−.20***	−.10*	
	Opportunity Risk	−.07**	.21		−.05*	.10	
	Behavior Risk	−.27***	−.17*		−.08**	−.09	
4	Protection-by-Risk Interactions			.005			.014*
	Controls Protection × Opportunity Risk		.12*				
	Controls Protection × Models Risk					.17**	
	Controls Protection × Vulnerability Risk					.09*	
	Models Protection × Opportunity Risk					.10*	
	Total R^2			.35			.16

N = 1087 (US), 1368 (China). Only significant interactions are included in the final model
* $p \leq .05$; ** $p \leq .01$; *** $p \leq .001$. All ΔR^2 and R^2 values are significant at $p \leq .001$
[a]Unstandardized regression weights of standardized predictor measures; standardized weights are inappropriate with interaction terms (see Aiken & West, 1991, pp. 40–47)
[b]Variance accounted for uniquely by protective factors = .09*** (US), .08*** (China)

had significant regression coefficients in relationship to the problem behavior criterion (MPBI), in either country sample, now have relatively large regression coefficients, while the Controls Protection measure, the major protective factor for the MPBI, does not, and it is not even significant in the China sample. This is a markedly different pattern.

The risk factor measures (models, vulnerability, opportunity, behavior), entered at Step 3, provided a very modest increment in variance accounted for (3 %, US; 1 %, nonsignificant, China). Noteworthy in this part of the analysis is that the Models Risk measure, which was the major risk factor for the problem behavior criterion (MPBI), is no longer significantly related, in either country sample, to the pro-social behavior criterion (MPSBI). Only the risk factor measure of Vulnerability Risk has a significant regression weight in the final regression model in both samples, and Behavior Risk is also significant in the US sample, as noted earlier. Finally, the twelve protection-by-risk interactions were tested for significance at Step 4. In the US sample, Controls Protection moderated Opportunity Risk; in the China sample, Controls Protection was a significant moderator of Models Risk, as noted earlier, and also of Vulnerability Risk, and Models Protection also moderated Opportunity Risk in the China sample.

In a supplemental hierarchical regression analysis, when the protective factors were entered after the risk factors, they accounted uniquely for 9 % (US) and 8 % (China) of variance, considerably more than the risk factors had (3 and 1 %, as noted above). All together, the entire set of theoretical predictor measures accounted for 35 % of the variance in pro-social behavior involvement in the US sample, and 16 % in the China sample, again a substantial and theoretically informative account—although less than that obtained for the measure of problem behavior involvement (48 and 39 %, respectively).

Discussion

The theoretical approach engaged in this study, Problem Behavior Theory, is a psychosocial explanatory framework developed over the past half century to provide understanding of adolescent and young adult behavior and development (Jessor et al., 1968; 1991; Jessor & Jessor, 1977; Jessor, 1991; 2014).

The protective and risk factors articulated in Problem Behavior Theory have, in the present study, provided substantial accounts of variation in both problem behavior and pro-social behavior, accounts that are largely parallel in pattern for adolescents in the US and the China samples. Those accounts have revealed that, although the protection measures and the risk measures make equivalent contributions to explaining problem behavior variation, protection makes a much larger contribution than risk when explaining variation in pro-social behavior. They have also made apparent the very different contributions that particular protective and risk factors make when accounting for problem behavior than when accounting for pro-social behavior. Together these findings call for a more nuanced understanding of the role of protection and risk in general and, more specifically, of the varying roles of particular protective and risk factors. It hardly makes sense any longer to speak of protective or risk factors as having certain impacts; it seems necessary, instead, to speak of their impacts in specific relationship to particular criteria or outcomes—in the present case, to either adolescent problem behavior or adolescent pro-social behavior.

The part played by protective factors in the present analyses is especially worth emphasizing. It challenges the overriding concern with risk and risk reduction that characterizes so much of current problem behavior research and intervention efforts and argues for a more balanced inclusion of the contribution that protection can make. Not only equivalent to the risk factors in their direct impact on problem behavior, the protective factors also emerged from this study as having effects as moderators or buffers of the impact of exposure to risk, Controls Protection moderating Models Risk in both country samples as the key example. Equally important, protective factors far outweighed risk factors in unique variance accounted for when predicting pro-social behavior, supporting its promotive as well as its preventive function. And involvement in pro-social behavior itself, the MPSBI measure, served as a significant protective factor against problem behavior in the US sample, although not in the China sample.

The important role of Controls Protection in regulating problem behavior in this study is consonant with the literature (e.g., Barber & Xia, 2013). On the other hand, Support Protection (analogous to the protective factor of "connectedness" in the literature) did not emerge as significant for problem behavior variation in either country sample, and this finding is consistent with results from an earlier wave of our data (Costa et al., 2005). It is also consonant with the results of Madkour et al., (2012) in their cross-national study of early sexual initiation in nine European countries: the negative association of parental support with early sexual initiation disappeared when parental knowledge (an indicator of Controls Protection) was added to the model. Support Protection *was* significant, however, and in both country samples, in predicting the positive criterion of pro-social behavior. These latter findings suggest the need for a more differentiated view of support/connectedness as a protective factor for problem behavior versus for pro-social behavior.

While the literature has largely been concerned with controls and connectedness, a contribution of the present study is the articulation of additional theoretically important protective and risk factors in the same systematic framework: Models Protection and Behavior Protection, and Models Risk, Vulnerability Risk, and Opportunity Risk, all of which contributed significantly to the explanatory account for one or both criterion measures. Indeed, Vulnerability Risk, an individual-level measure, emerged as a significant predictor for both problem behavior and pro-social behavior. Clearly, further theoretical articulation can still be achieved in the quest for a more comprehensive account. For one example, there is a theoretically promising contextual construct, "Opportunity Protection." Although it was not assessed in this study, it would be a logically relevant addition to the explanatory scheme in future research.

The pattern of significant protective and risk factor predictors that emerged in Table 11.3 changed markedly and similarly in both country samples, when the criterion measure shifted, in Table 11.4, from problem behavior (MPBI) to pro-social behavior (MPSBI); this shift is a key finding of the present study. From its pre-eminent role among the protective factors in predicting problem behavior (Table 11.3), Controls Protection shifts to a relatively minor and even insignificant (for China) role when the criterion is pro-social behavior (Table 11.4). Likewise, Models Protection and Support Protection, neither protective factor significant in the final model accounting for problem behavior in the US and China samples (Table 11.3), become the two major protective factor predictors when the criterion shifts to pro-social behavior (Table 11.4), and they are, indeed, the only protective factors that are significant in the China sample. Turning to the risk factors, a similar marked shift in pattern can be seen, and in both country samples, with the shift in outcome criterion predicted from problem to pro-social behavior. Models Risk, which had the largest *b* coefficient when predicting problem behavior, is no longer even a significant risk factor when accounting for pro-social behavior. These findings are important in illuminating the varying roles that a particular protective or risk factor may play depending on what the predictive focus is. Their different implications for efforts to reduce problem behavior versus to promote positive behavior would seem to deserve serious attention.

The inclusion of Behavior Protection, the MPSBI measure, as a protective factor when predicting involvement in problem behavior, and of Behavior Risk, the MPBI measure, as a risk factor when predicting involvement in pro-social behavior follows from the theoretical position that actual involvement or experience with particular behaviors has an impact on the likelihood of engaging in other behaviors, both conventional and unconventional. Engaging in heavy drinking, for example, has implications for engaging in smoking and for lesser involvement with parents than with peers; on the other hand, involvement with, say, religion has implications for engaging in other conventional or pro-social activities and for avoiding problem behavior involvement. Nevertheless, the issue of endogeneity can be raised since those behavioral predictors are themselves the outcome of the other protective or risk factors in the Problem Behavior explanatory scheme. To address this issue, we re-ran the regression analyses in Tables 11.3 and 11.4, omitting the Behavior Protection measure from Table 11.3 and the Behavior Risk measure from Table 11.4. The results were essentially the same. The proportion of variance accounted for remained almost identical, and the overall pattern of findings with the behavior predictors omitted is pervasively congruent with the findings reported in Tables 11.3 and 11.4.

The robustness of the results obtained in this study can be made apparent in several ways. First, the analysis of the Wave-3 problem behavior criterion in Table 11.3 can be compared with the results from the comparable analysis of the Wave-1 data reported in an earlier paper (Jessor et al., 2003). Findings were pervasively similar across the two different waves of data thus supporting the replication of the Problem Behavior Theory model at both the early- and the mid-adolescent developmental stages in accounting for problem behavior.

Another approach to appraising the robustness of the problem behavior findings was an analysis that controlled for the contribution of the individual-level measures [Attitudinal Intolerance of Deviance (a component of Controls Protection); Behavior Protection; Vulnerability Risk; and Behavior Risk], and that sought to determine whether the MPBI findings held for the social context measures of protection and risk alone, i.e., when individual-level measures as well as socio-demographic measures were controlled. The results of that analysis (table available from the authors) are fully consonant with the explanatory model as a whole: Controls Protection and Models Risk were still the most important protection and risk measures, respectively, both in their main effects and in their interaction. Of further interest from that analysis, the social context measures of the protective and risk factors were, taken together, able to account for substantial variance in problem behavior involvement

(19 %, US; 17 %, China), with socio-demographic and individual-level measures controlled. This latter point is of special interest because of the linkage of protective and risk factors in the literature to the concept of "resilience." The tendency to ascribe resilience to the individual, as a personal characteristic, has been widespread, but as several key investigators have noted: "Resilience… does not represent a personality trait or an attribute of the individual" (Luthar & Cicchetti, 2000, p. 857); and "resilience may reside in the social context as much as within the individual" (Rutter, 1993, p. 626). Our finding that social context protective and risk factors alone can account for substantial problem behavior variance supports the view that resilience is as much an outcome of processes in the environment of daily adolescent life as it is of processes in the adolescent.

Finally, the comparable pattern of findings observed across the two country samples further attests to the robustness of the explanatory framework, a framework at the underlying genotypic level, even when applied to samples that are descriptively so different and drawn from such diverse societies. As argued in a recent commentary (Jessor, 2008), genotypic generality often underlies phenotypic specificity in cross-national inquiry.

Several limitations constrain inferences about the findings of this study. First, the present findings represent relationships that have been observed at a particular time, and causal inferences are not warranted. It is the case, however, that in our earlier studies of developmental change in a different positive outcome, an index of health-enhancing behavior (Turbin et al., 2006; Jessor et al., 2010), change in protective and risk factors over time was shown to be predictive of change in the health-enhancing behavior index over both a 1-year and a 2-year interval. Second, it is possible that the relative contributions of protection and risk reported in the analyses could simply reflect differential adequacy or comprehensiveness of measurement. The fact is, however, that the protective factor variables and the risk factor variables were all based on multiple-item scales with good reliability (Table 11.1), and both the problem and the pro-social behavior measures, the MPBI and the MPSBI, were multi-item indexes.

There are additional limitations, as well. A third limitation needing acknowledgement is that the data are all self-report. In earlier reports from the larger study, however, it was possible to compare a subsample of adolescent Wave-1 reports of their perceived social contexts with independent reports about those same contexts by their parents. "Those comparisons revealed a significant degree of consistency. providing some indication of. external validity" (Turbin et al., 2006, p. 453). Fourth, it should be clear that the samples employed in the present study, drawn from local, urban, school-based settings, cannot in any way represent the countries from which they were drawn; rather, they constitute similar samples from countries and settings known to be different on a variety of dimensions, from economic system to family structure to traditional values. Finally, the differential retention rate between Wave-1 and Wave-3 in the two country samples (71 %, US; 87 %, China) might have affected the results through differential loss of the more problem-prone adolescents; such loss, however, is more likely to affect mean scores on problem behavior than the underlying theoretical relationships among the variables involved.

Conclusion

The Problem Behavior Theory framework of protective and risk factors has received impressive support from the findings in this study. The analyses of two contrasting outcome criteria—problem behavior and pro-social behavior—have contributed to a more differentiated perspective about protection and risk as explanatory constructs for understanding *both* problem and pro-social behavior in adolescence. That the very same protective or risk factor plays a different role when different outcome criteria are engaged has emerged as a novel and important finding. Although Controls Protection was the pre-eminent protective factor in accounting for problem behavior in both country samples, it was only modestly related to pro-social behavior in the US sample and not related at all in the China sample. Likewise, neither Models Protection nor Support Protection was related significantly to problem behavior in either country sample, but both were highly significant predictors of pro-social behavior. Important also is the evidence for the positive or promotive role of protective factors in relationship to pro-social behavior as well as their preventive role in relationship to problem behavior.

Together, the findings not only strengthen the Problem Behavior Theory framework but they advance the kind of understanding about protection and risk that can usefully inform the design of intervention efforts. Hopefully, the study makes clear the advantages that would accrue to both the problem behavior constituency and the positive youth development constituency if each engaged *both* problem behavior and pro-social behavior in future research on adolescent behavior and development. The antinomy between those two research constituencies has long ago lost its warrant.

Acknowledgments Data collection was supported by William T. Grant Foundation (Grant No. 99202099).

References

Aiken, L. S., & West, S. G. (1991). *Multiple regression: Testing and interpreting interactions*. Newbury Park, CA: Sage.

Barber, B. K. (1997). Introduction: Adolescent socialization in context—the role of connection, regulation, and autonomy in the family. *Journal of Adolescent Research, 12*(1), 5–11.

Barber, B. K., & Olsen, J. A. (1997). Socialization in context: Connection, regulation, and autonomy in the family, school, and neighborhood, and with peers. *Journal of Adolescent Research, 12*(2), 287–315.

Barber, B. K., & Xia, M. (2013). The centrality of control to parenting and its effects. In R. E. Larzelere, A. S. Morris, & A. W. Harrist (Eds.), *Authoritative parenting: Synthesizing nurturance and discipline for optimal child development* (pp. 61–87). Washington, DC: American Psychological Association.

Benson, P. L. (1997). *All kids are our kids*. San Francisco: Jossey-Bass.

Bernat, D. H., Oakes, J. M., Pettingell, S. L., & Resnick, M. (2012). Risk and direct protective factors for youth violence: Results from the National Longitudinal Study of Adolescent Health. *American Journal of Preventive Medicine, 43*(2), S57–S66.

Blum, R. W., Halcon, L., Beuhring, T., Pate, E., Campell-Forrester, S., & Venema, A. (2003). Adolescent health in the Caribbean: Risk and protective factors. *American Journal of Public Health, 93*(3), 456–460.

Ciairano, S., et al. (2009). Adolescent risk behavior in Italy and The Netherlands: A cross-national study of psychosocial protective factors. *European Psychologist, 14*(3), 180–192.

Cohen, J. (1990). Things I have learned (so far). *American Psychologist, 45*(12), 1304–1312.

Costa, F. M., Jessor, R., Turbin, M. S., Dong, Q., Zhang, H., & Wang, C. (2005). The role of social contexts in adolescence: Context protection and context risk in the U.S. and China. *Applied Developmental Science, 9*, 67–85.

Guerra, N. G., & Bradshaw, C. P. (2008). Linking the prevention of problem behaviors and positive youth development: Core competencies for positive youth development and risk prevention. In N. G. Guerra & C. P. Bradshaw (Eds.), *Core competencies to prevent problem behaviors and promote positive youth development. New directions for child and adolescent development* (Vol. 122, pp. 1–17). Hoboken, NJ: Wiley.

Hawkins, J. D., Catalano, R. F., & Miller, J. Y. (1992). Risk and protective factors for alcohol and other drug problems in adolescence and early adulthood: Implications for substance abuse prevention. *Psychological Bulletin, 112*(1), 64–105.

Herrenkohl, T. I., Lee, J., & Hawkins, J. D. (2012). Risk versus direct protective factors and youth violence: Seattle Social Development Project. *American Journal of Preventive Medicine, 43*(2), S41–S56.

Hilliard, L. J., Bowers, E. P., Greenman, K. N., Herschberg, R. M., Geldof, G. J., Glickman, S. A., et al. (2014). Beyond the deficit model: Bullying and trajectories of character virtues in adolescence. *Journal of Youth and Adolescence*. doi:10.1007/s10964-014-0094-y.

Jessor, R. (1991). Risk behavior in adolescence: A psychosocial framework for understanding and action. *Journal of Adolescent Health, 12*(8), 597–605.

Jessor, R. (2008). Description versus explanation in cross-national research on adolescents. *Journal of Adolescent Health, 43*(6), 527–528.

Jessor, R. (2014). Problem Behavior Theory: A half-century of research on adolescent behavior and development. In J. Brooks-Gunn, R. M. Lerner, A. C. Petersen, & R. K. Silbereisen (Eds.), *The developmental science of adolescence: History through autobiography*. New York: Psychology Press.

Jessor, R., Donovan, J. E., & Costa, F. M. (1991). *Beyond adolescence: Problem behavior and young adult development*. New York: Cambridge University Press.

Jessor, R., Graves, T. D., Hanson, R. C., & Jessor, S. L. (1968). *Society, personality, and deviant behavior: A study of a tri-ethnic community*. New York: Holt, Rinehart and Winston.

Jessor, R., & Jessor, S. L. (1977). *Problem behavior and psychosocial development: A longitudinal study of youth*. New York: Academic Press.

Jessor, R., Turbin, M. S., & Costa, F. M. (1998a). Protective factors in adolescent health behavior. *Journal of Personality and Social Psychology, 75*(3), 788–800.

Jessor, R., Turbin, M. S., & Costa, F. M. (1998b). Risk and protection in successful outcomes among disadvantaged adolescents. *Applied Developmental Science, 2*, 194–208.

Jessor, R., Turbin, M. S., & Costa, F. M. (2010). Predicting developmental change in healthy eating and regular exercise among adolescents in China and the United States: The role of psychosocial and behavioral protection and risk. *Journal of Research on Adolescence, 20*(3), 707–725.

Jessor, R., Turbin, M. S., Costa, F. M., Dong, Q., Zhang, H., & Wang, C. (2003). Adolescent problem behavior in China and the United States: A cross-national study of psychosocial protective factors. *Journal of Research on Adolescence, 13*(3), 329–360.

Jessor, R., Van Den Bos, J., Vanderryn, J., Costa, F. M., & Turbin, M. S. (1995). Protective factors in adolescent problem behavior: Moderator effects and developmental change. *Developmental Psychology, 31*(6), 923–933.

Kerr, M., & Stattin, H. (2000). What parents know, how they know it, and several forms of adolescent adjustment: Further support for a reinterpretation of monitoring. *Developmental Psychology, 36*(3), 366–380.

Knight, G. P., & Hill, N. E. (1998). Measurement equivalence in research involving minority adolescents. In V. C. McLoyd & L. D. Steinberg (Eds.), *Studying minority adolescents: Conceptual, methodological, and theoretical issues* (pp. 183–210). Mahwah, NJ: Lawrence Erlbaum Associates.

Lerner, R. M., & Benson, P. L. (Eds.). (2003). *Developmental assets and asset-building communities: Implications for research, policy, and practice*. New York: Kluwer.

Lewin, K. (1935). *A dynamic theory of personality: Selected papers*. New York: McGraw-Hill.

Lösel, F., & Farrington, D. P. (2012). Direct protective and buffering protective factors in the development of youth violence. *American Journal of Preventive Medicine, 43*(2), S8–S23.

Luthar, S. S., & Cicchetti, D. (2000). The construct of resilience: Implications for interventions and social policies. *Development and Psychopathology, 12*(4), 857–885.

Madkour, A. S., Farhat, T., Halpern, C. T., Gabhainn, S. N., & Godeau, E. (2012). Parents' support and knowledge of their daughters' lives, and females' early sexual initiation in nine European countries. *Perspectives on Sexual and Reproductive Health, 44*(3), 167–175.

Madkour, A. S., Farhat, T., Halpern, C. T., Godeau, E., & Gabhainn, S. N. (2010). Early adolescent sexual initiation as a problem behavior: A comparative study of five nations. *Journal of Adolescent Health, 47*(4), 389–398.

McClelland, G. H., & Judd, C. M. (1993). Statistical difficulties of detecting interactions and moderator effects. *Psychological Bulletin, 114*(2), 376–390.

Ndugwa, R. P., Kabiru, C. W., Cleland, J., Beguy, D., Egondi, T., Zulu, E. M., et al. (2010). Adolescent problem behavior in Nairobi's informal settlements: Applying Problem Behavior Theory in sub-Saharan Africa. *Journal of Urban Health, 88*(Suppl. 2), 298–317.

Pardini, D. A., Loeber, R., Farrington, D. P., & Stouthamer-Loeber, M. (2012). Identifying direct protective factors for nonviolence. *American Journal of Preventive Medicine, 43*(2), S28–S40.

Phelps, E., Balsano, A. B., Fay, K., Peltz, J. S., Zimmerman, S. M., Lerner, R. M., et al. (2007). Nuances in early adolescent developmental trajectories of positive and problematic/risk behaviors: Findings from the 4-H study of positive youth development. *Child and Adolescent Psychiatric Clinics of North America, 16*, 473–496.

Piko, B. F., & Kovacs, E. (2010). Do parents and school matter? Protective factors for adolescent substance use. *Addictive Behaviors, 35*(1), 53–56.

Rutter, M. (1993). Resilience: Some conceptual considerations. *Journal of Adolescent Health, 14*(8), 626–631.

Simantov, E., Schoen, C., & Klein, J. D. (2000). Health-compromising behaviors: Why do adolescents smoke or drink? Identifying underlying risk and protective factors. *Archives of Pediatrics and Adolescent Medicine, 154*(10), 1025–1033.

Turbin, M. S., Jessor, R., Costa, F. M., Dong, Q., Zhang, H., & Wang, C. (2006). Protective and risk factors in health-enhancing behavior among adolescents in China and the United States: Does social context matter? *Health Psychology, 25*(4), 445–454.

Vazsonyi, A. T., Chen, P., Jenkins, D. D., Burcu, E., Torrente, G., & Sheu, C.-J. (2010). Jessor's Problem Behavior Theory: Cross-national evidence from Hungary, the Netherlands, Slovenia, Spain, Switzerland, Taiwan, Turkey, and the United States. *Developmental Psychology, 46*(6), 1779–1791.

Vazsonyi, A. T., Chen, P., Young, M., Jenkins, D., Browder, S., Kahumoku, E., et al. (2008). A test of Jessor's Problem Behavior Theory in a Eurasian and a Western European developmental context. *Journal of Adolescent Health, 43*(6), 555–564.

Chapter 12
Some Concluding Thoughts

Richard Jessor

As the chapters in this volume make plain, it has been a long journey from the origins of Problem Behavior Theory in the Tri-ethnic Community Study of the early 1960s to its current formulation nearly six decades later. The theory that has evolved is best schematized in Fig. 12.1, various versions of which have appeared in our publications since the mid-1990s.

Unpacking the Conceptual Framework

Several aspects of the current representation of Problem Behavior Theory in Fig. 12.1 warrant review. First, the breadth of behavioral relevance of the theory is apparent; it has by now encompassed the domains of adolescent/young adult problem behavior, health-enhancing behavior, and pro-social behavior. While instantiations of behaviors in each domain are shown in the Figure, they are intended as illustrative only and not meant to be exhaustive. Each behavior shown in the Figure has been engaged in our studies over the years, as well as various others not listed there.

Second, all three behavior domains are boxed together in the Figure in order to indicate that they are interrelated, that is, that there is co-variation between domains as well as within domains. Co-variation within the problem behavior domain is well established and has been captured by our widely used concept of a problem behavior *syndrome*. Co-variation within the other domains has also been empirically established in our work, as has co-variation between all three domains.

R. Jessor (✉)
Institute of Behavioral Science, University of Colorado at Boulder, Boulder, CO 80309, USA
e-mail: jessor@Colorado.edu

R. Jessor, *The Origins and Development of Problem Behavior Theory*,
Advancing Responsible Adolescent Development,
DOI 10.1007/978-3-319-40886-6_12

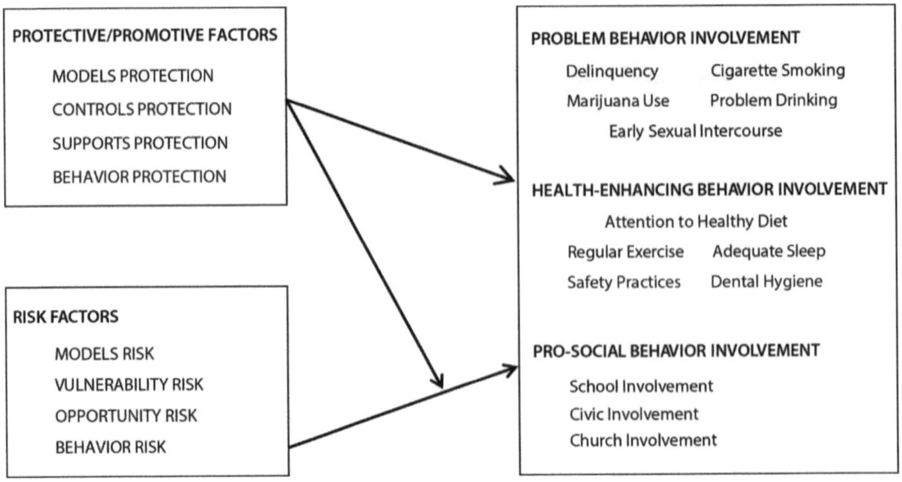

Fig. 12.1 Problem Behavior Theory explanatory model for adolescent risk behavior

Such co-variation has implications for the organization of individuality, of the way an adolescent or young adult is in the world, i.e., of a *lifestyle*, a concept about behavioral organization we have found more useful than a focus on any of the separate behaviors in isolation.

Third, the theoretical determinants of the behavioral domains are differentiated into either *protective/promotive* factors or *risk* factors, and four types of each have been articulated. Each type has been shown in our research to be significantly related to variation in the behavioral domains. It is important, again, not to see these four types of risk and of protective/promotive factors as exhaustive; they are simply those we have engaged in our research. Other sources of risk and protection are worth examining; one we are especially interested in exploring in future research would be called Opportunity Protection, referring to access to resources and favorable circumstances, which we expect to be of special importance in promoting positive, pro-social behavior.

Fourth, the essential dynamic in Problem Behavior Theory is the dialectic between protective/promotive factors (the upper arrow) and risk factors (the lower arrow), and their interaction (the middle arrow). Risk factors increase the likelihood of involvement in risk behavior and lessen the likelihood of involvement in pro-social or health-enhancing behavior; protective/promotive factors, by contrast, prevent or limit involvement in risk behavior and increase the likelihood of involvement in pro-social or health-enhancing behavior. The interaction of protection and risk moderates the impact of exposure to risk and, thereby, buffers the influence that risk factors can have on involvement in risk behavior.

Fifth, the dialectic is founded on fundamental social learning theory processes that underlie engaging in any behavior or in behavior change: *models* for learning and practicing the behavior (social learning); *supports* (rewards) for engaging in it; *controls* (sanctions) against engaging in it; and *having already engaged in a behavior* that is connected to or implicates a new behavior (e.g., having already begun smoking is a behavior that is connected in the social learning ecology with initiating drinking).

Sixth, it is important to emphasize again that the theory engages *both person and context*, that is, both the individual and his/her social environment. All of the behavior measures in the Figure are assessed at the individual level; also assessed at the individual level are such psychosocial measures as Intolerance of Deviance (a measure of Controls Protection), and Low Self-Esteem, Low Perceived Life Chances, Low Expectations for Academic Achievement, and Depression (measures of Vulnerability Risk). All the other measures of Models, Controls, Supports, and Opportunity in the Figure involve assessments of the social context of daily adolescent/young adult life.

Finally, it is essential in using this theoretical model that its measures reflect the larger context in which it is applied. An assessment of, say, Models Risk for drinking, should reflect the entirety of drinking models in the adolescent's social ecology, e.g., family models for drinking, peer models for drinking, school models for drinking, neighborhood models for drinking, media models for drinking. Assessed in this comprehensive way, the theoretical constructs in Problem Behavior Theory have yielded substantial accounts of variation in adolescent and young adult behavior, both problem and pro-social.

Risk Behavior as Part of Normal Development

The samples used in our decades of research, despite their diversity in age, gender, regional, national, or international context, or in periods of historical time, have all been drawn from the normal population. This approach has supported a perspective about adolescent risk behavior as part of normal development, a perspective that is at odds with those perspectives—sometimes based on clinical samples or samples at the extremes of involvement in risk behavior—that invoke notions of psychopathology, or have recourse to medical concepts of disease, or that reduce explanation to ideas about the immaturity or pathology of the brain. Although possibly applicable to such unrepresentative or extreme samples, these latter perspectives seem to us gratuitous at best and misleading at worst. As our research findings have shown across the decades, substantial explanation of adolescent/young adult risk behavior—often accounting for as much as half the variance—is provided by social–psychological theory that views risk behavior as socially learned, socially supported, and socially and personally controlled. The research has also shown that risk behaviors are functional and that engaging in them can serve normal developmental goals, e.g., expressing independence from parents, gaining respect from peers, rejecting the values and expectations of conventional society, and perhaps most important, signaling a transition to a more mature status, e.g., smoker, drinker, nonvirgin. The warrant for explanatory recourse to psychopathology, or to disease, or to the immature brain seems to be based more on the disciplinary proclivities of medicine and psychiatry or the reductive impulses of psychology than on the robustness of the social science evidence.

The Relative Influence of Protective/Promotive Factors Versus Risk Factors

Research on adolescent problem behavior and, indeed, on the larger field of adolescent risk behavior, has been dominated historically by a preoccupation with risk and risk reduction. Although attention to protection and protective factors has increased in recent decades, protection is still most often invoked as just another approach to reducing risk. What has been elided in such an interpretation of protection is the fact that protective factors, in addition to reducing risk, can have a *promotive* effect on engaging in positive, pro-social behavior, as well. That is the contribution that protective factors can make when risk is absent, or when the objective is to enhance positive youth development. Throughout our research with both risk factors and protective factors, we have found that, when the concern is with problem behavior, risk factors and protective factors account for similar proportions of the explained variance. However, when the behavioral criterion to be explained is a positive one, e.g., pro-social behavior or health-enhancing behavior, then protective factors account for far more of the variance than do risk factors. That is because, beyond their protective function (against risk), they have a promotive function as well, and it is this promotive function that was demonstrated in Chap. 11. The implications of such theorizing and such findings are that far more attention needs to be paid to protection and to articulating protective/promotive factors in adolescent/young adult research, and that increased attention to protective/promotive factors is a way to bridge the current divide between the risk-oriented problem behavior constituency and the promotion-oriented positive youth development constituency.

Key Protective Factors and Key Risk Factors for Prevention/ Intervention

Although there has been much emphasis in the literature on the role of social support in problem behavior prevention, our findings have yielded a more nuanced understanding of its role and of the roles played by the other protective and risk factors. In relation to problem behavior prevention, it is actually *controls protection*, both personal and social, that is most important, and *support protection* plays only a minimal role. When the intervention concern is with enhancing pro-social behavior, however, that is when support protection becomes important, as does models protection, with controls protection now playing only a minimal role. Among the risk factors, it is models risk that is most important in regard to problem behavior, but it plays only a minimal role in relation to enhancing pro-social behavior. Thus *the intervention objective matters*; for promoting positive, pro-social behavior, support protection and models protection become key; for reducing problem behavior, controls protection and lessening models risk become key. Obviously, the most salutary and comprehensive intervention approach would engage both kinds of key protective and risk factors, aiming simultaneously to reduce problem behavior while promoting pro-social behavior.

Risk Behavior Versus Risk-Taking Behavior

Driving an automobile involves a significant amount of risk of having an accident, yet we don't refer to people who drive cars as "risk takers" or their driving as "risk-taking behavior." Unfortunately, that understanding is widely violated in accounts of adolescent involvement in the variety of problem behaviors that put them at risk; those behaviors are often termed "risk-taking" behaviors, and adolescents are, thereby, often labelled as "risk takers." As pointed out in Chap. 8, this terminological stance is the source of considerable explanatory mischief. The tautology that stems from defining problem behaviors, or risk behaviors more generally, as risk-taking behaviors, and adolescents as risk takers, offers only circular reasoning rather than explanation. Clearly, behaviors such as smoking, or drug use, or drinking, or early or unprotected sex, or sedentary behavior entail risk for health, development, relations with parents, encounters with the law, etc. They warrant, therefore, the term "risk behaviors" because engaging in them entails the possibility of negative consequences or health- or life-compromising outcomes. But with few exceptions—such activities as drag racing or rock climbing or skydiving, perhaps, in which there is the deliberate taking of risk for the excitement and thrill of managing the danger—problem behaviors are not usually engaged in for the thrill of managing their possible negative outcomes, e.g., the thrill of being able to avoid pregnancy or a sexually transmitted disease by engaging in unprotected sex. Defining adolescents as risk takers and risk behaviors as risk-taking behaviors fails to advance understanding and forestalls the quest for a more comprehensive and illuminating account. It would be salutary for developmental science if the "risk taking" term were abandoned and were replaced by the term "risk behavior" instead.

The Dimension of Conventionality–Unconventionality

The Problem Behavior Theory account of adolescent problem behavior over the decades has illuminated an important, social–psychological dimension of variation among adolescents relevant to their involvement in problem behavior. We have described it as a dimension of *conventionality–unconventionality*, characterizing both the adolescent and the adolescent's immediate social context. In general terms, it refers to the degree to which the adolescent is committed to the norms and institutions of conventional society—parents/family, school, church, civic organizations—and is embedded in—bonded to—those institutions. Ties to family, commitment to school and its academic goals, engagement with church or other community organizations all combine to orient the adolescent toward supporting the norms of conventional society. Lesser involvement entails an orientation away from conventional society and its institutions of authority toward supporting peer norms and values and, more recently, toward the influences of social media, instead. Many of the measures that operationalize the risk factor and protective/promotive factor constructs in Problem Behavior Theory tend to reflect location along the conventionality–unconventionality dimension. For example, friends' models for academic achievement versus friends' models for drinking, or support from parents or teachers versus support from peers reflect the conventionality–unconventionality contrast in the adolescent's social context; at the person level, for example, high versus low tolerance of deviance, a personal control, reflects that same dimension. It is useful, in relation to accounting for variation in involvement in problem or risk behavior or variation in the developmental earliness-lateness of its initiation, to consider the adolescent's location on the social–psychological dimension of conventionality–unconventionality.

A Final Note

The chapters in this volume offer a window on both process and product. The product is the current formulation of Problem Behavior Theory, and the process has been the revisions and extensions of the conceptual framework as it evolved through successive empirical tests of its explanatory reach. As a social–psychological approach, the theory has yielded consistent illumination about young people, their behavior, their development and, indeed, their lives, across differences in age, gender, location—whether local, national, or international—and historical time. My hope is that this volume will help make Problem Behavior Theory more accessible and available to researchers around the world. Toward that end, I am also providing the web site for the 32-page, theory-derived *Adolescent Health and Development Questionnaire* (AHDQ) which is the most recent instrument we have used to assess the concepts in the theory:

http://www.colorado.edu/ibs/jessor/questionnaires/questionnaire_ahdq3.pdf

Finally, despite the usefulness of Problem Behavior Theory documented in the selections in this book, so much more remains to be established about how young people grow up, especially under circumstances of disadvantage and limited resources and even danger. As with all social science, the challenge of exhaustive explanation remains elusive. My hope is that other scholars and researchers will go further and deeper than we have in telling the story about how young people, though engaging in risk behavior, nevertheless find a way to flourish.

Index

R. Jessor, *The Origins and Development of Problem Behavior Theory*,
Advancing Responsible Adolescent Development,
DOI 10.1007/978-3-319-40886-6

MIX
Papier aus verantwortungsvollen Quellen
Paper from responsible sources
FSC® C105338

If you have any concerns about our products,
you can contact us on
ProductSafety@springernature.com

In case Publisher is established outside the EU,
the EU authorized representative is:
Springer Nature Customer Service Center GmbH
Europaplatz 3, 69115 Heidelberg, Germany

Printed by Libri Plureos GmbH
in Hamburg, Germany